PILATES

WITH WORKOUT CIRCLE

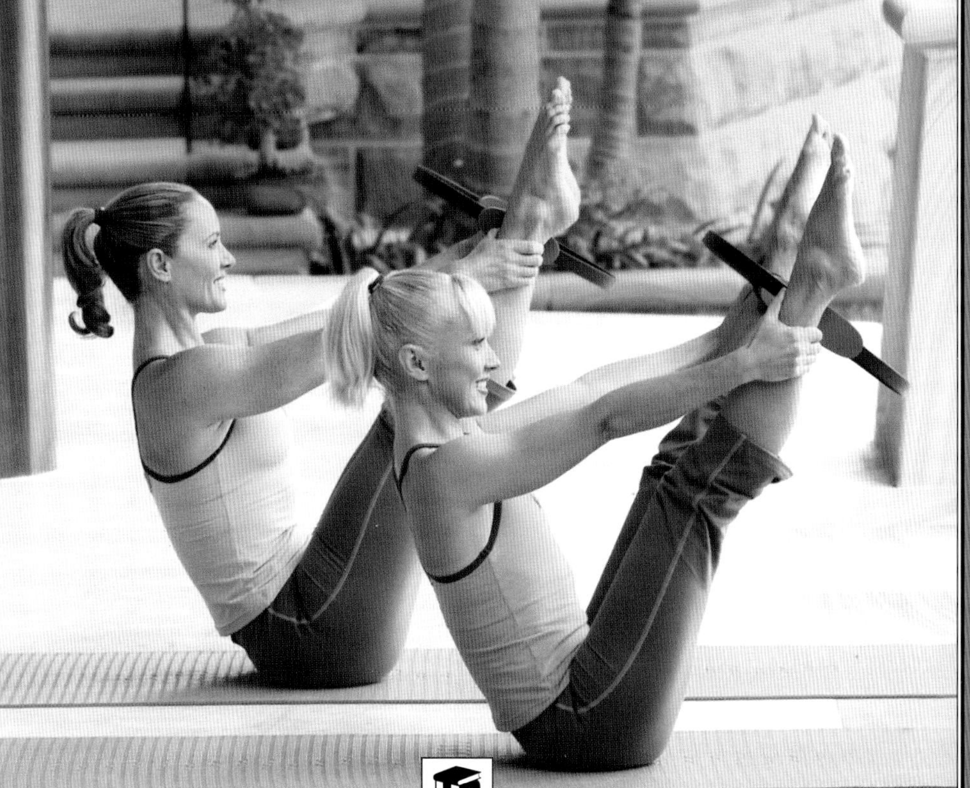

HINKLER BOOKS

Authors: Dina Matty and Keft Burdell
Art Director: Karen Moores
Editor: Carol Campbell
Graphic Artist: Susie Allen
Photographer: Paul Broben

First published in 2006
by Hinkler Books Pty Ltd
45–55 Fairchild Street
Heatherton Victoria 3202 Australia
www.hinklerbooks.com

2 4 6 8 10 9 7 5 3
07 09 11 10 08

Printed and bound in China

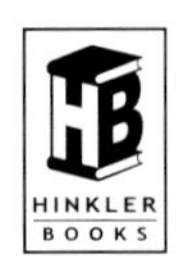

ISBN-10: 1 7415 7790 X
ISBN-13: 978 1 7415 7790 7

Contents

INTRODUCTION

Joseph H Pilates was a German-born fitness expert, who, in the early 1900s, designed a system of exercises that combined stretching and strengthening using apparatus with spring resistance and mat exercises. He described it as 'contrology', or the art of control, which encompassed six principles: concentration, control, centring, precision, breathing and flow.

Today, the Pilates Method of body conditioning has become world renowned and has a successful record of creating healthy, balanced bodies along with additional benefits, which include:

- lengthened muscles
- improved posture
- preventing and healing injuries
- improved flexibility
- having fun while working out
- enhanced energy and rejuvenation.

Pilates with Workout Circle is an extension of a basic/intermediate mat workout with modified progressions.

Here we introduce the workout circle – a piece of equipment from the Pilates system that adds an additional challenge. It is important, therefore, to integrate it gradually into your workout. You should complete the full mat sequence first, without the workout circle, because this, in itself, is an intermediate level mat workout. The exercises are based on the original sequence as taught by Joseph Pilates, so they should be followed in the same order unless you have injuries, in which case you should modify each exercise as specified. Once you have achieved this level, start to incorporate the workout circle into the first six exercises. And then gradually add it into the other mat exercises at your own pace. This workout should eventually take up to 30 minutes.

The workout circle enhances the intensity of the exercise and offers many additional benefits, including:

- a greater and deeper connection to your powerhouse
- working your inner/outer thighs and glutes
- strengthening your arms
- strengthening your whole body.

REQUIREMENTS

During your Pilates floor workout, ensure you have a comfortable surface to lie on, one that is neither too hard nor too soft. A mat is ideal. In some exercises you might need a small pillow to place beneath your head to alleviate tension in your neck and shoulder muscles. Have a low chair or stool close by for seated exercises.

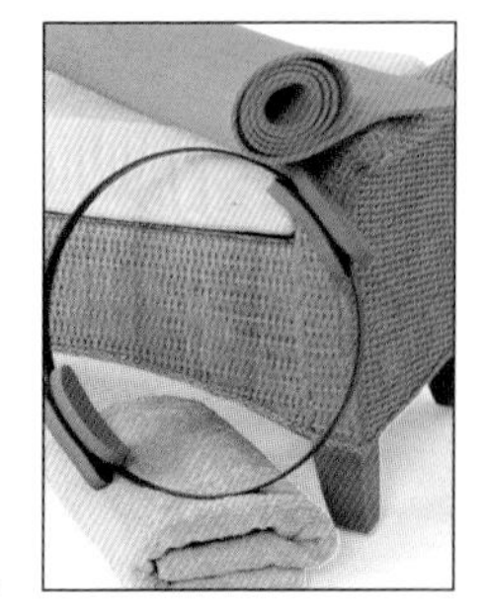

At all times, remember to apply the principles of stretch, strength and control, and enjoy increased feelings of wellbeing and an improved quality of life.

Elements of a Pilates Workout

The Powerhouse

All of the work in Pilates comes from your powerhouse, which is the band of muscle that wraps around your torso. It also includes your bottom and inner and outer thighs.

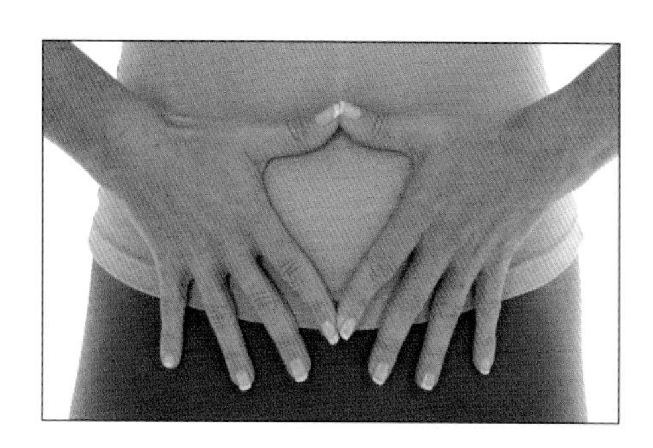

Closing the Rib Cage

At this intermediate level become aware of your rib cage. For example, in the Roll-Up, when your arms are extended over your head, keep your ribs on the mat and imagine drawing your rib cage down towards your hips, so that your upper back presses down into the mat and doesn't arch.

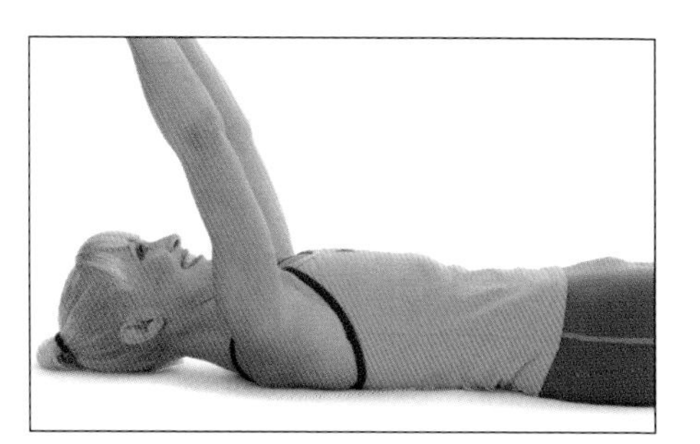

Pilates Stance

In Pilates with Workout Circle, you work in Pilates stance, with your heels together and toes slightly apart. This enables your glutes to work, rather than your quadriceps.

Breathing

How you breathe is a key part of a Pilates workout. It is important to inhale through your nose and exhale through your mouth. As you inhale, imagine you are expanding your back on the mat. As you exhale, draw your ribs together and draw the navel to the spine.

The Pilates Principles

The mat work with the workout circle encompasses the following six Pilates principles.

Concentration

Focus and visualise throughout the workout to help connect your mind and body.

Control

Use concentration and control to help achieve the ultimate goal of each exercise.

Centring

All the work on the Pilates mat comes from your centre, or powerhouse.

Precision

Perform each individual movement on the mat with precision.

Breathing

Controlled breathing enables you to perform with quality of movement.

Flow

The sequence of the mat is performed in a smooth flowing movement. Each movement should be fluid with dynamic energy.

Positioning the Workout Circle

When using the workout circle, never put it directly on to a joint.

When used between your legs, place the workout circle just above your ankle bone on the fleshy part of your leg.

When holding the workout circle with your arms, keep your fingers long and relaxed with the workout circle on the heels, or lower palms of your hands (all fingers and thumbs on the same side).

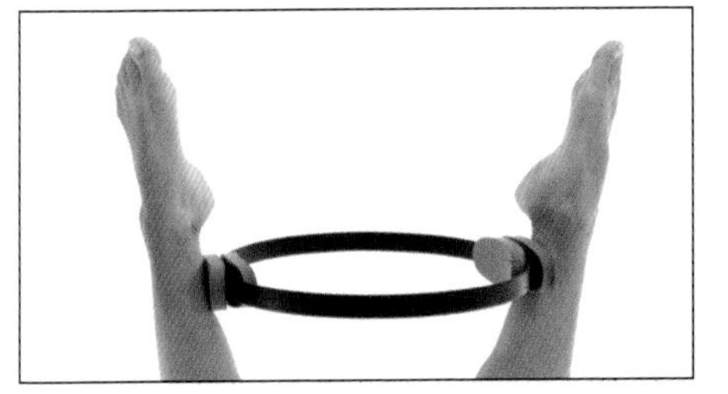

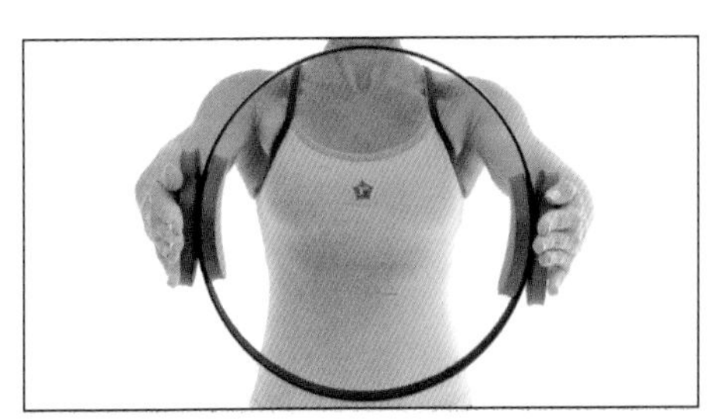

Workout Circle Preparation

1 Lie on your back, feet hip-width apart, knees bent.

2 Place the workout circle on your inner thigh, just above your knees. Keep hands by your sides.

3 Inhale. As you exhale scoop in, engage your bottom and try to squeeze the workout circle from your bottom and inner thighs. If you can't feel your bottom engaging, place your fingertips on the back of your thighs and try again. Think of scooping your belly in, squeezing your bottom and then squeezing the workout circle. Your goal is to change the shape of the circle.

4 Repeat 5–8 times.

Note

To prevent injury while working through your workout circle exercises, it is important to feel the squeeze through your bottom, and not your knees.

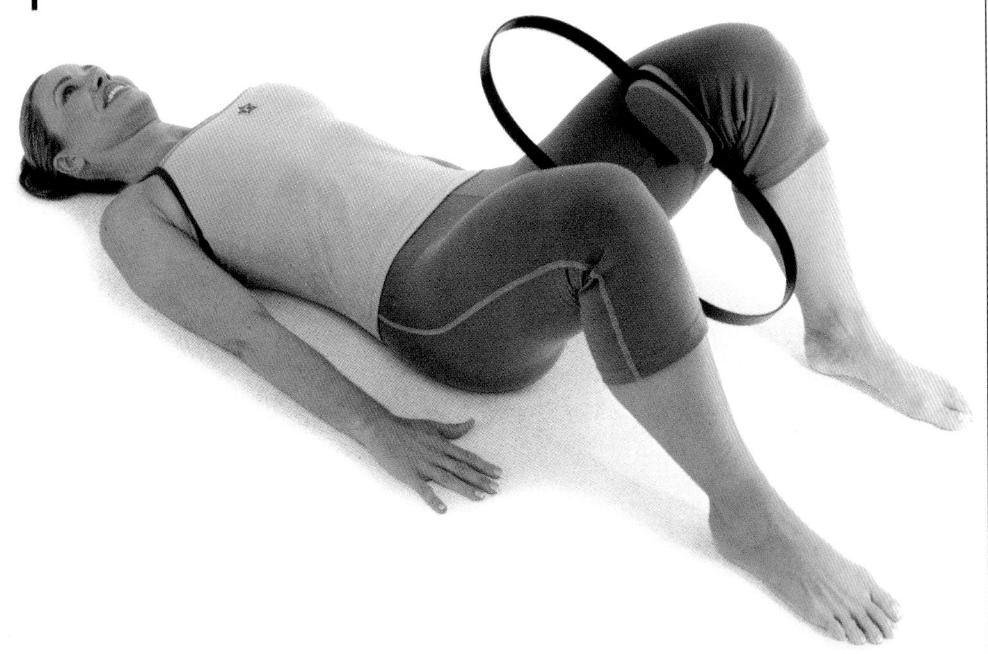

The Hundred

A warm-up and breathing exercise to increase circulation and enhance endurance.

1 Lie on your back, drawing your knees into your chest. Place the workout circle between your ankles (just above the ankle bone), draw your chin to your chest and extend arms forward reaching from your armpits. Extend legs towards the ceiling, wrapping your thighs around and engaging the workout circle. Lower your legs to where you can feel your powerhouse engage (but not that low that your back arches off the mat).

2 Begin to pump your arms and inhale through your nose for five counts; exhale through your mouth for five counts, at the same time scooping in through your powerhouse and keeping the workout circle engaged throughout. This is one set of 10; continue until you have reached 100.

3 Bend your knees into your chest and take the workout circle in your hands. Extend your legs out on to the mat and take the workout circle overhead ready for the Roll-Up.

Note

Make sure you are using your powerhouse and glutes to engage the workout circle, and not your knees.

If you feel any pain in your lower back, lift your legs higher towards the ceiling, or bend your knees, or try it without the workout circle.

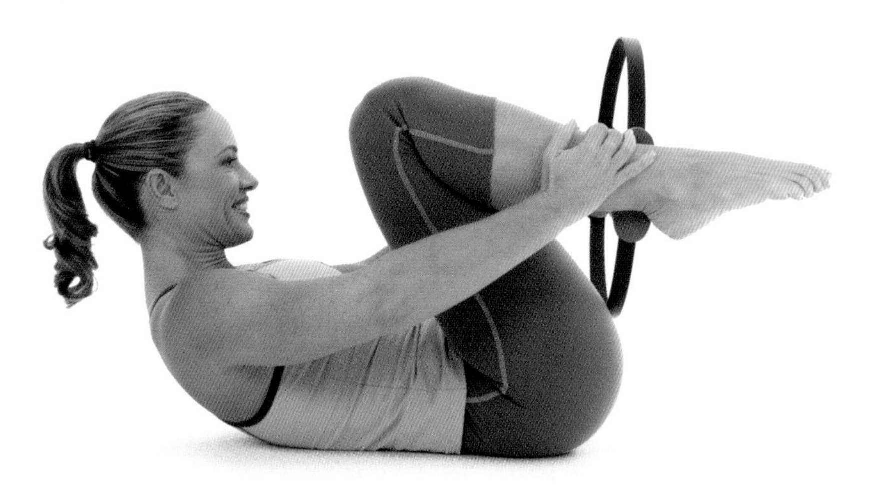

Modifications

Neck problems: Use a pillow and lower your head if straining your neck.

Lower back problems: As you progress through the Pilates program your powerhouse will strengthen and your lower back pain may decrease, but you can always modify the exercise by bending your knees throughout the mat workout.

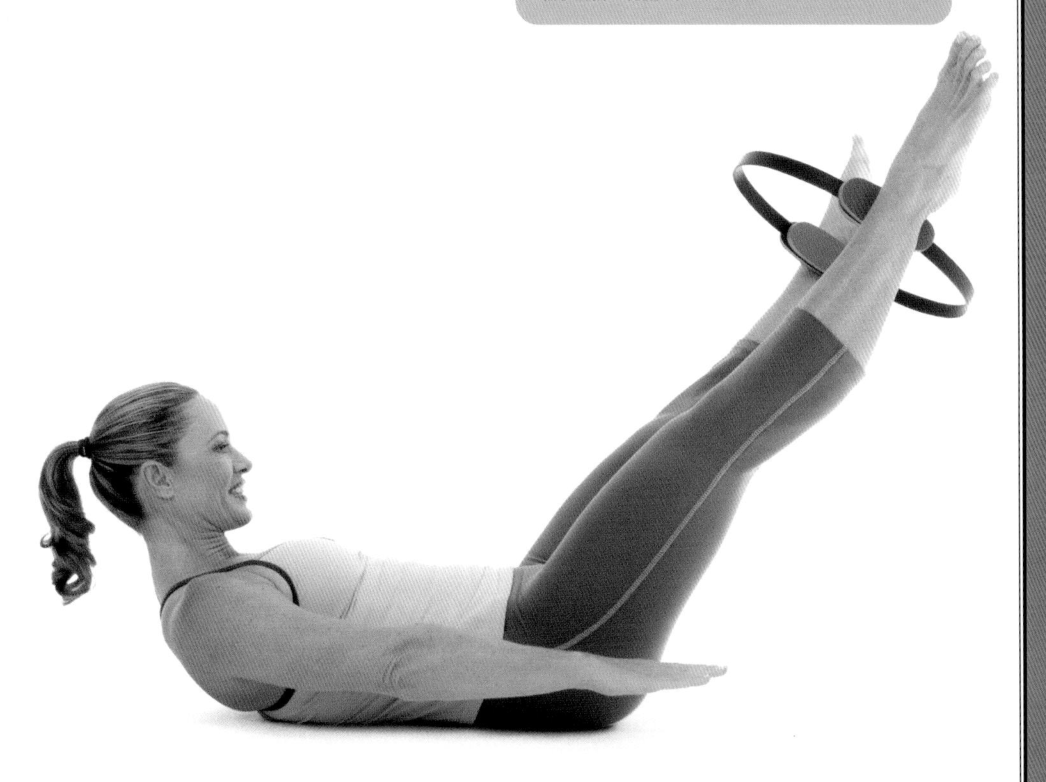

THE ROLL-UP

Strengthens your powerhouse, articulates your spine and stretches your hamstrings.

1 Lie on your back. Holding the workout circle with the heel of your hands, stretch your arms over your head, keeping your fingers long and making sure the whole of your spine is imprinted on to the mat and your ribs are closed.

2 Raise your arms to the ceiling and bring your chin to your chest, lightly pressing the heel of your hands into the workout circle. Look through the window of your arms. Inhale, scoop in and roll up, keeping the workout circle engaged so you can scoop in deeper. Exhale as you reach forward, maintaining the C-curve.

3 Inhale and pull in deeper, keeping the workout circle engaged, as you peel your spine back on to the mat. Exhale as you stretch your arms over your head.

4 Repeat 4 times.

MODIFICATIONS

Lower back/disc problems: Keep your knees bent at a 45-degree angle to ease the pressure on your lower back.

Knee problems: Try to maintain a soft knee when your legs are extended.

NOTE

Place the workout circle to one side and walk your hands up your legs if you are not quite strong enough to roll up.

Keep your shoulders relaxed and try not to lock your elbows when squeezing the workout circle.

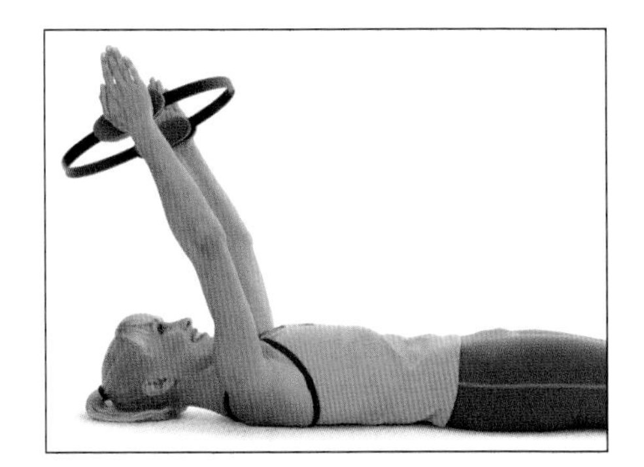

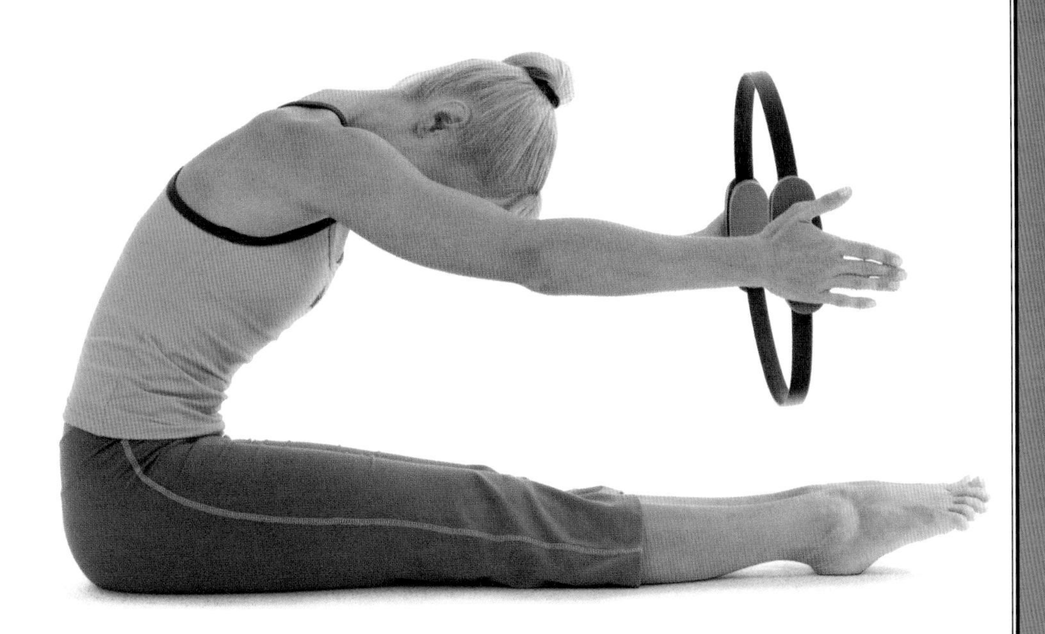

Single-Leg Circles

Stretches and strengthens the leg in the hip joint and stabilises the pelvis.

This exercise does not include the workout circle.

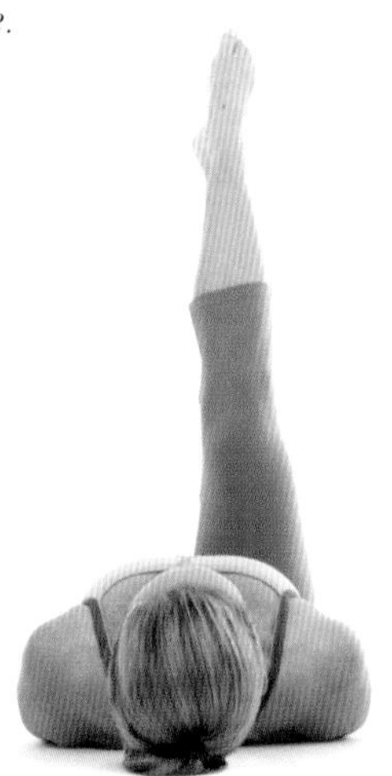

1 After the last roll-up, place the workout circle by your side on the mat.

2 Lie on your back and extend your right leg to the ceiling. Walk your hands up your leg and, depending on your flexibility, hold your thigh, calf or ankle.

3 Bring your chin to your chest and exhale, stretching your leg towards your nose.

4 Place your head back down with your arms by your sides. Scoop in and leave your leg in the air, wrapping your thigh so your bottom is engaged and the quadriceps relaxed.

5 Maintaining stability in your hips, scoop in and reach your leg across your body, 'drawing' a circle on the ceiling, and then coming back towards your nose.

6 Repeat 4 times and then reverse the circle, maintaining hip stability and the scoop. Scissor your legs to change and repeat on your other side, beginning with the stretch.

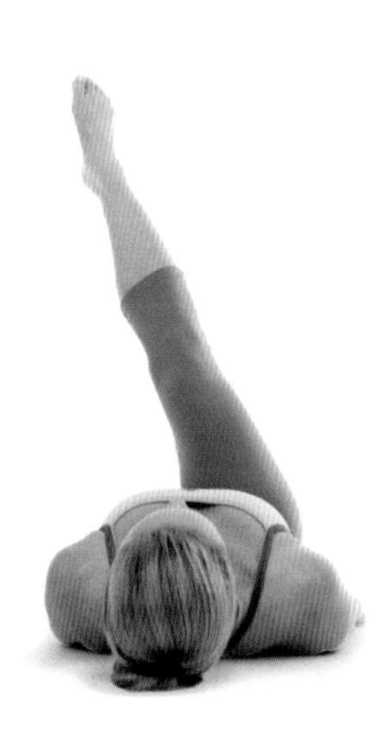

Note

Ensure you are using your powerhouse to control the circle of your leg.

If you can't maintain pelvic stability, draw a smaller circle in the air.

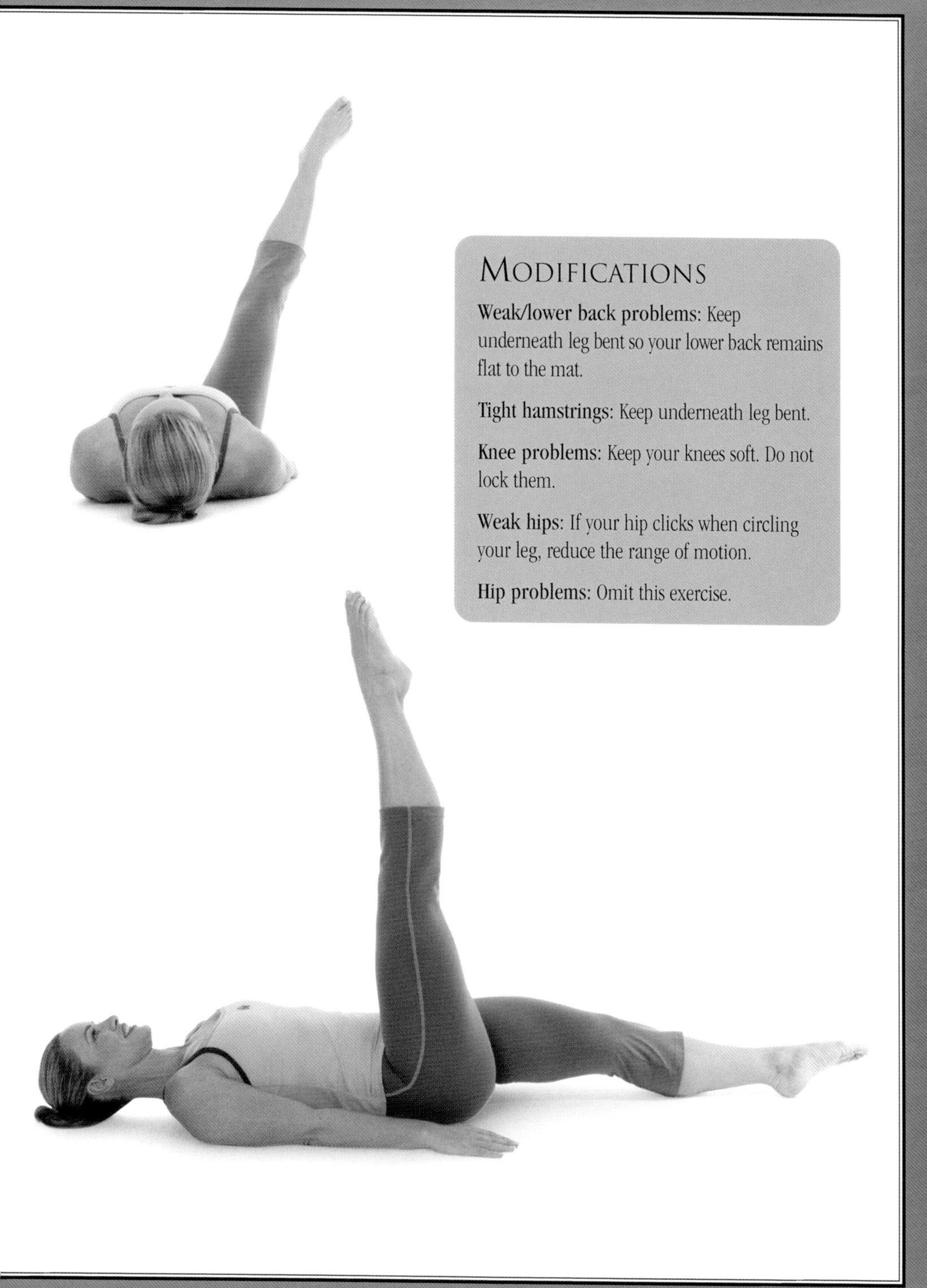

Modifications

Weak/lower back problems: Keep underneath leg bent so your lower back remains flat to the mat.

Tight hamstrings: Keep underneath leg bent.

Knee problems: Keep your knees soft. Do not lock them.

Weak hips: If your hip clicks when circling your leg, reduce the range of motion.

Hip problems: Omit this exercise.

Rolling Like a Ball

Works the powerhouse and massages the spine for balance and control.

1 Lower your leg after the last circle and roll up off the mat. Lift your hips and come forward to the front edge of your mat. Bend your knees into your chest. Place the workout circle between your ankles, wrapping your hands around the outside of your ankles (not holding the workout circle). During this exercise, ensure your ankles are kept in line with your hips. The squeeze of the workout circle comes from your inner thighs and bottom.

2 Bring your chin towards your chest and draw your nose down towards your navel. Scoop in and draw your toes up off the mat.

3 Inhale and roll back as you lift your hips up towards the ceiling. Squeeze the workout circle, scooping in deeper as you exhale and come forward to balance.

4 Repeat 4 times.

Note

Watch out that your knees don't roll inwards during this exercise. Ensure they remain in line with your ankles.

Make sure you use your bottom and inner thighs to squeeze the workout circle. Roll only as far as your shoulder blades.

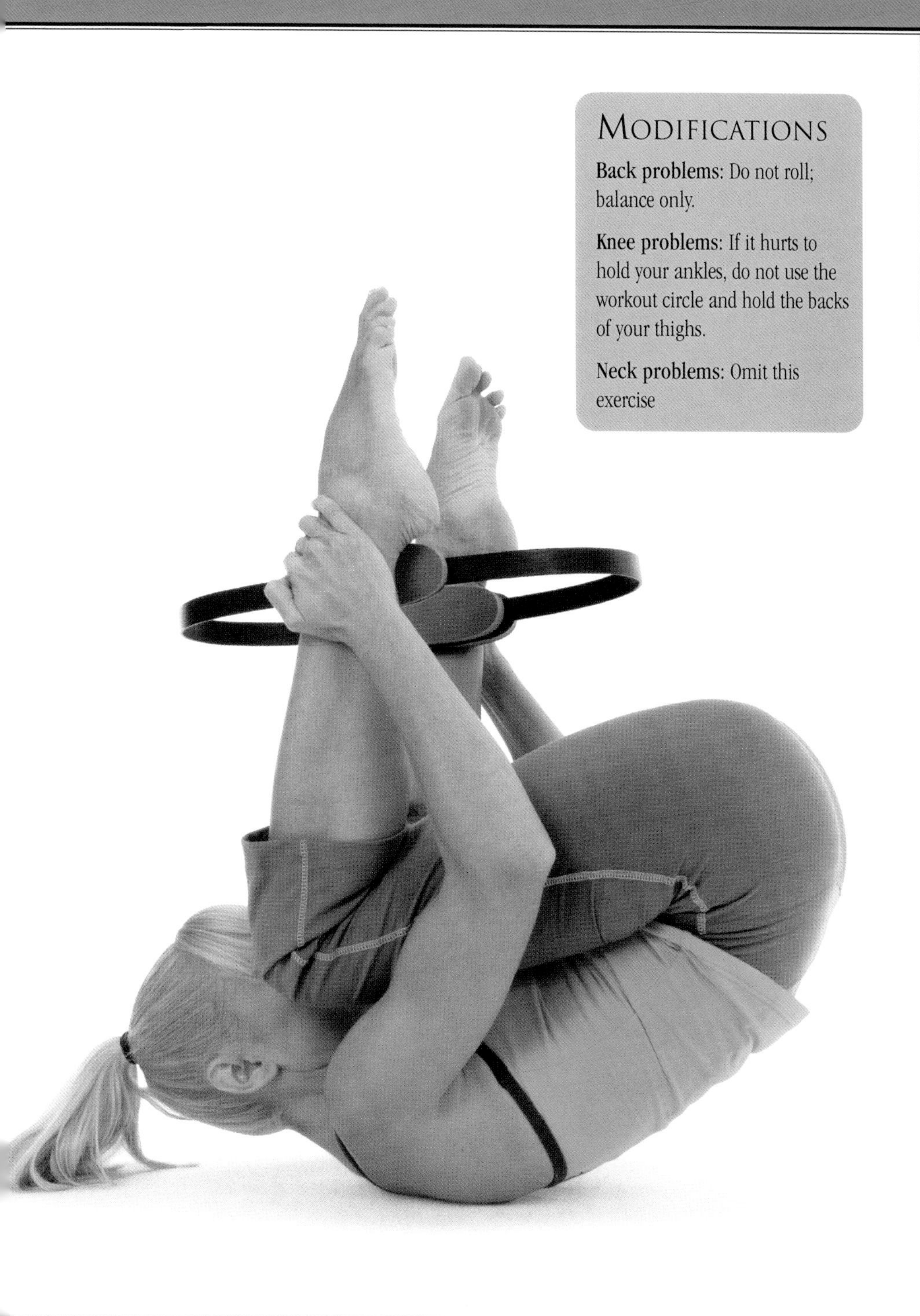

Modifications

Back problems: Do not roll; balance only.

Knee problems: If it hurts to hold your ankles, do not use the workout circle and hold the backs of your thighs.

Neck problems: Omit this exercise

Stomach Series

Five exercises that strengthen the powerhouse and increase flexibility.

Single-Leg Stretch

1 Place your toes down on to the mat and remove the workout circle. Slide back and lie down. Holding the workout circle with the heels of your hands, extend both arms forward.

2 Draw your right knee into your chest, extend your left leg forward off the mat at a 45-degree angle.

3 Inhale. Draw your left knee to your chest, right leg extended. Exhale. Change legs again, drawing your right knee into your chest, left leg extended.

4 Repeat 7 times.

5 Throughout this exercise, your back must remain flat on the mat, using your powerhouse to change legs and reaching the workout circle forward and up.

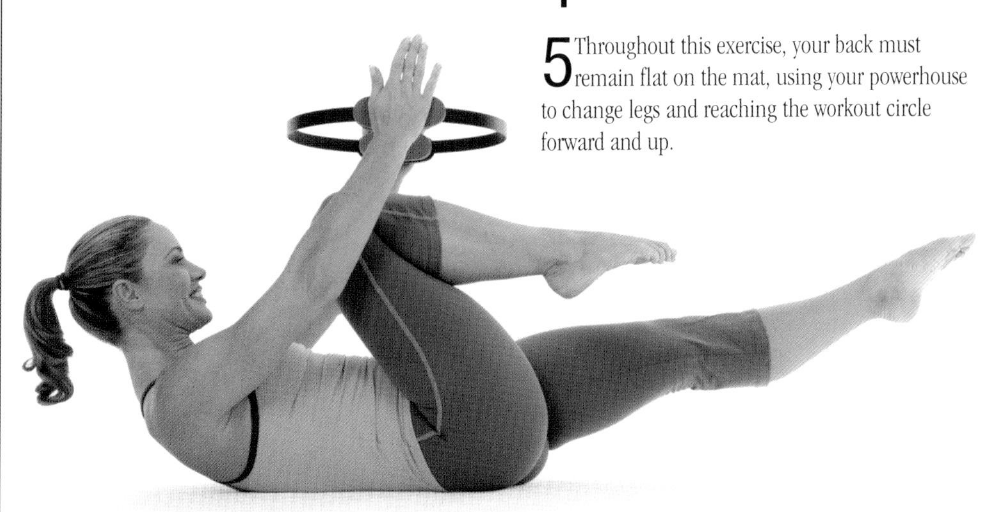

Note

Keep your chin glued to your chest and emphasise the scoop of your powerhouse to change legs.

Keep the base of your shoulder blades on the mat and draw your shoulders down into your back as you squeeze the workout circle.

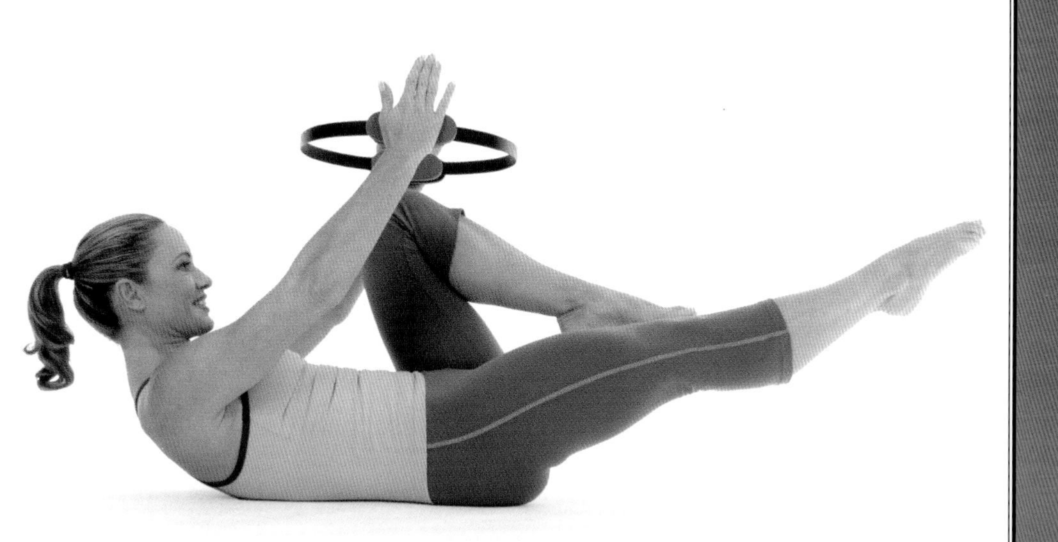

DOUBLE-LEG STRETCH

This exercise can be completed holding the workout circle between your hands, as for the Single-Leg Stretch, or between your ankles, as described here.

1 Draw both knees into your chest and place the workout circle just above your ankles. Part your knees slightly to open your lower back and place your hands on your ankles.

2 Inhale. Extend your arms so they are level with your ears, and extend your legs until they are at a 45-degree angle, squeezing the workout circle from your bottom.

3 Scoop in and exhale. Circle your arms back and around and draw your knees into your chest.

4 Repeat 7 times.

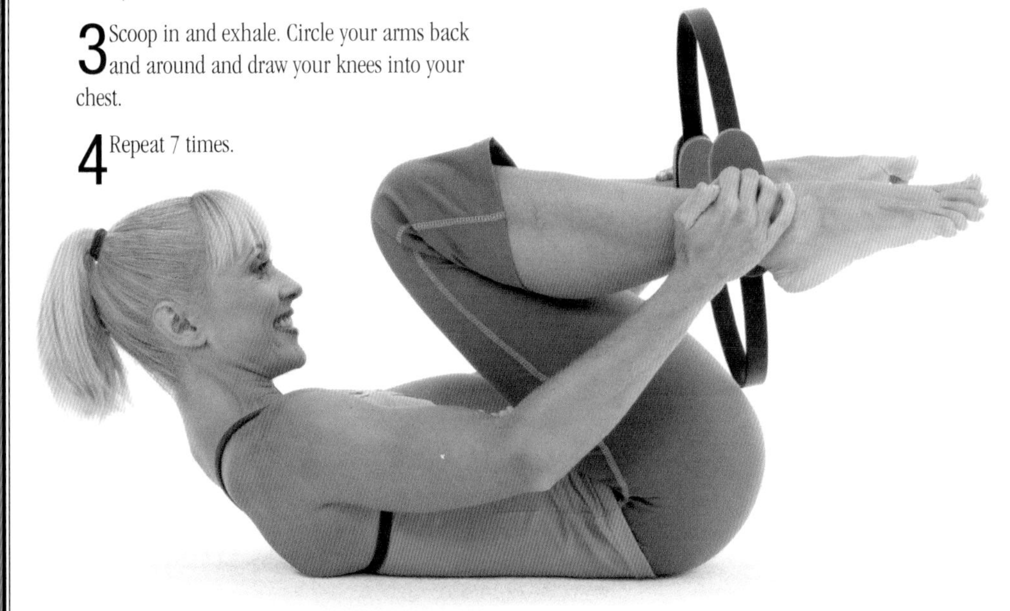

Note

When extending your legs make sure you are scooping in and your back is flat on the mat.

Do not use your knees to squeeze the workout circle, and make sure you are engaging from your bottom.

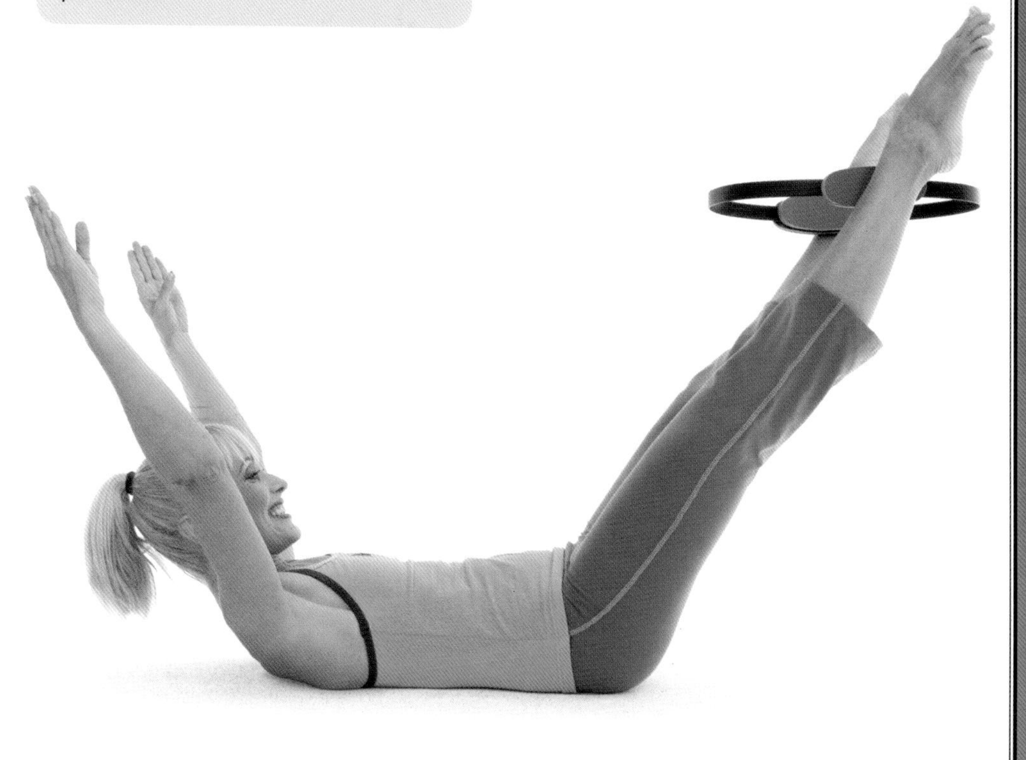

SINGLE-LEG STRAIGHT

This exercise does not include the workout circle.

1 Extend both legs towards the ceiling. Place your hands on the back of your thigh, calf or ankle, depending on your flexibility.

2 Lower your left leg and pulse your right leg twice towards your nose. Scissor your legs to change and repeat on the left. Make sure you scoop in your powerhouse when you pulse your leg.

3 Repeat 9 times.

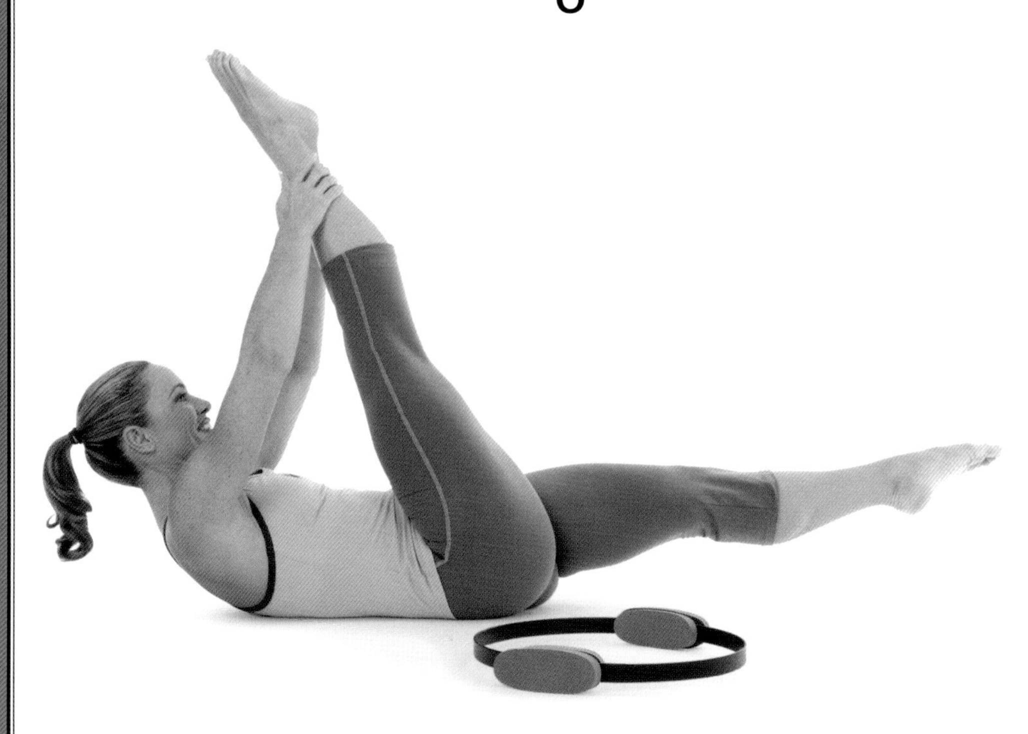

Note

Keep a nice rhythm during this exercise. Ensure you use your powerhouse to pulse your leg, rather than your arms, and keep your legs as straight as possible.

Try not to lift your shoulders off the mat. Try to maintain contact with the mat.

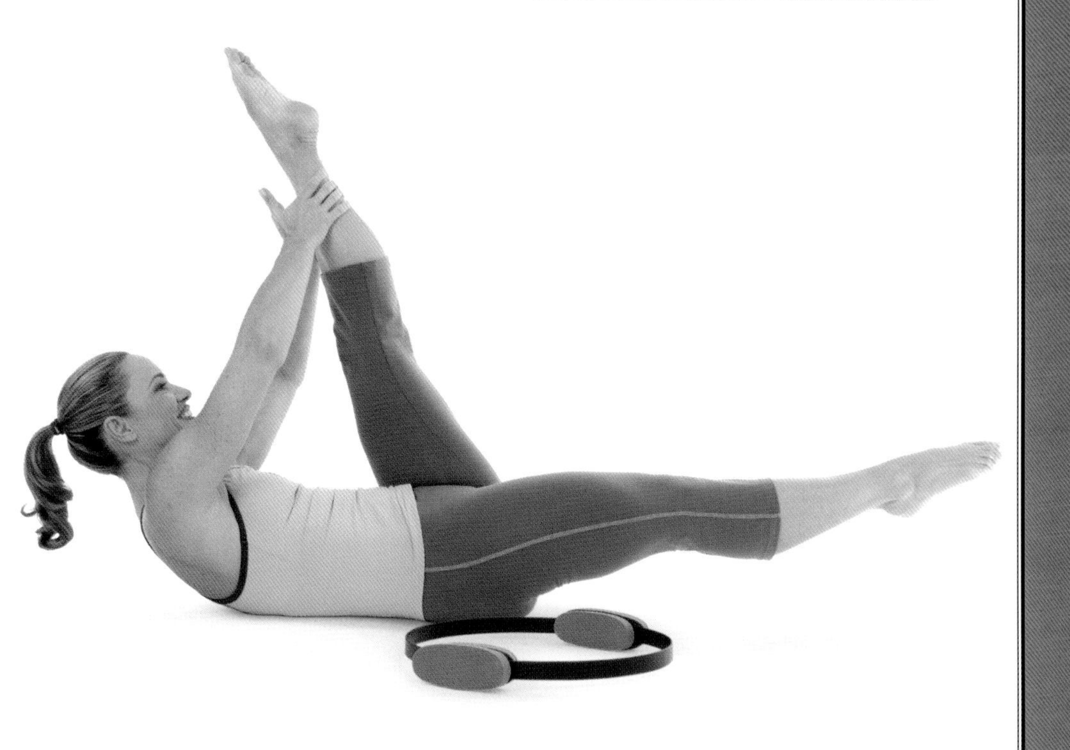

DOUBLE-LEG STRAIGHT

1 Begin by bringing both knees into your chest and place the workout circle just above your ankles. Put your hands behind your head, one hand on top of the other.

2 Extend your legs straight to the ceiling, squeezing the workout circle from your bottom and your inner thighs.

3 Inhale. Lower your legs, at the same time squeezing the workout circle from your bottom (ensuring your back stays flat).

4 Exhale. Scoop in deeper and use your powerhouse to draw your legs back up, keeping the workout circle engaged.

5 Repeat 5 times.

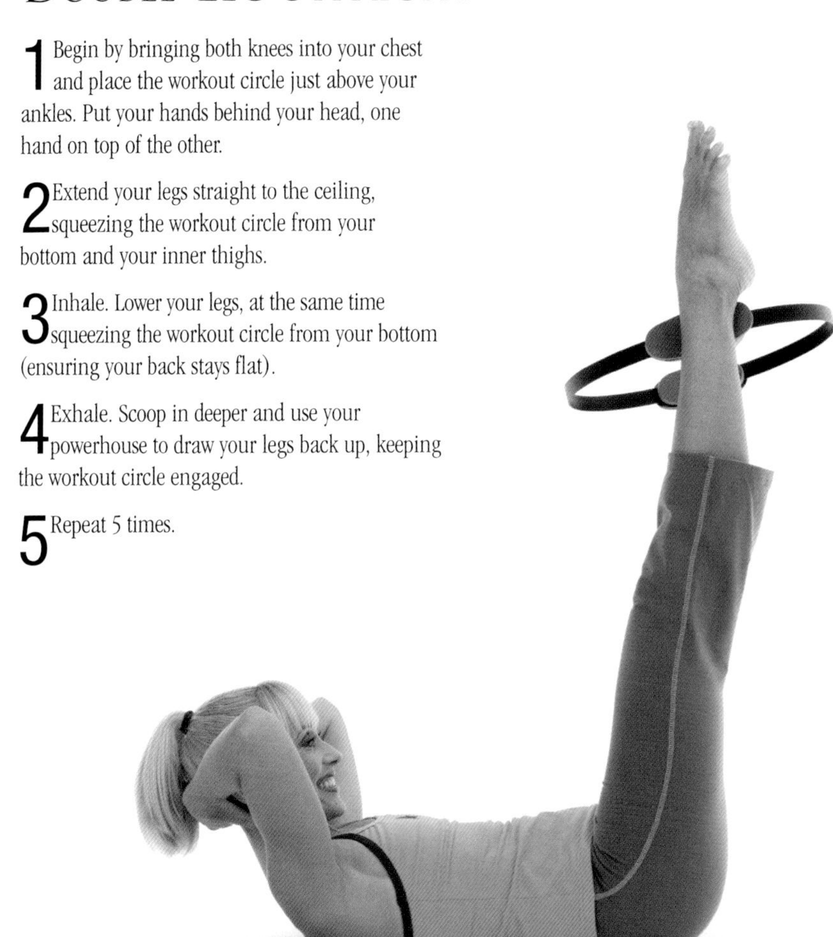

Note

Keep your chin to your chest. Squeeze your bottom to engage the workout circle and use your powerhouse, not your hip flexors, to draw your legs up.

If you feel any lower back pain, reduce the range of motion or bend your knees. If you still have pain, omit this exercise.

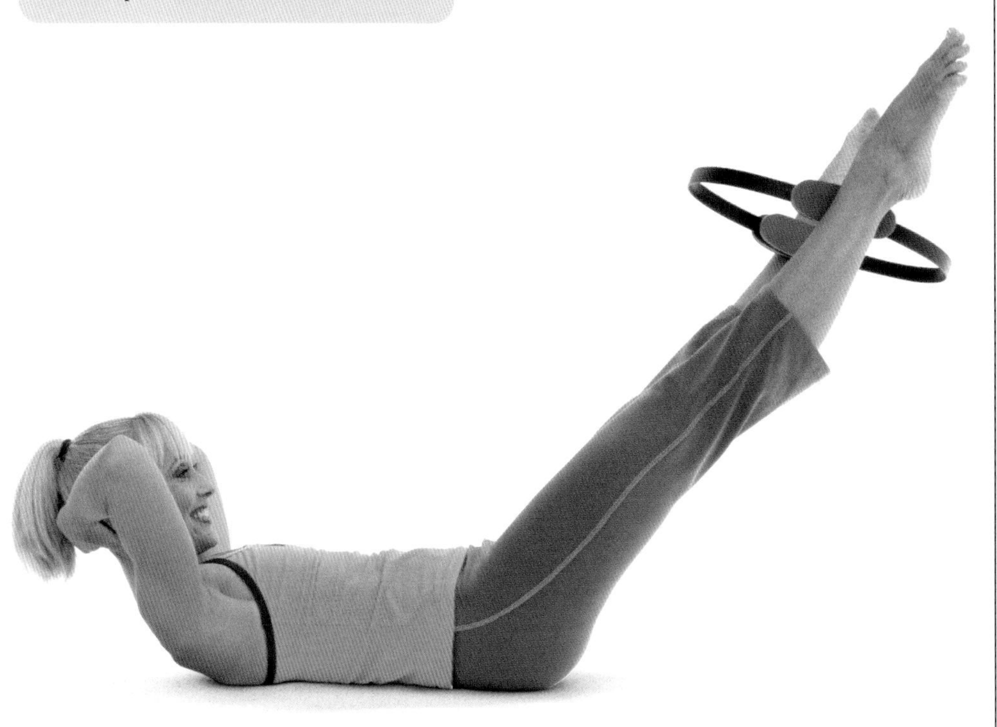

Criss-Cross

1 Begin with your knees brought into your chest. Keep your hands behind your head, chin to your chest and the workout circle still between your ankles.

2 Inhale as you extend both legs forward, and exhale as you twist your torso to the right, looking back towards your right elbow. Keep the workout circle engaged and lengthen out of your hips.

3 Inhale as your return to the centre, bending your knees into your chest. Exhale and extend your legs as you twist to the left.

4 Repeat once.

Note

Reach out of your hips when your legs are extended and keep your spine centred on the mat at all times, using your breath to twist.

Keep your legs at a 45-degree angle, with legs extended. As you twist, try not to let your lower back arch.

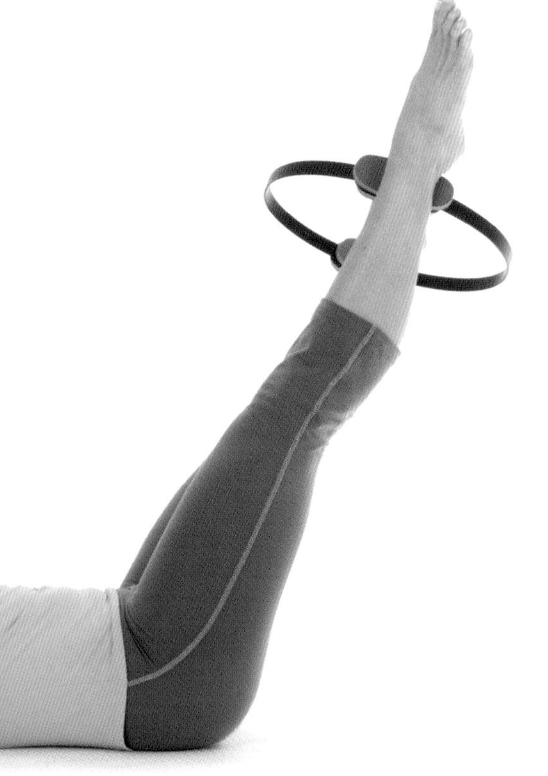

Modifications

Lower back problems: Keep your legs at a 45-degree angle, and use a small range of motion. Leave out twisting.

Neck problems: Try to keep your head up for half the exercise and then rest your head on a pillow.

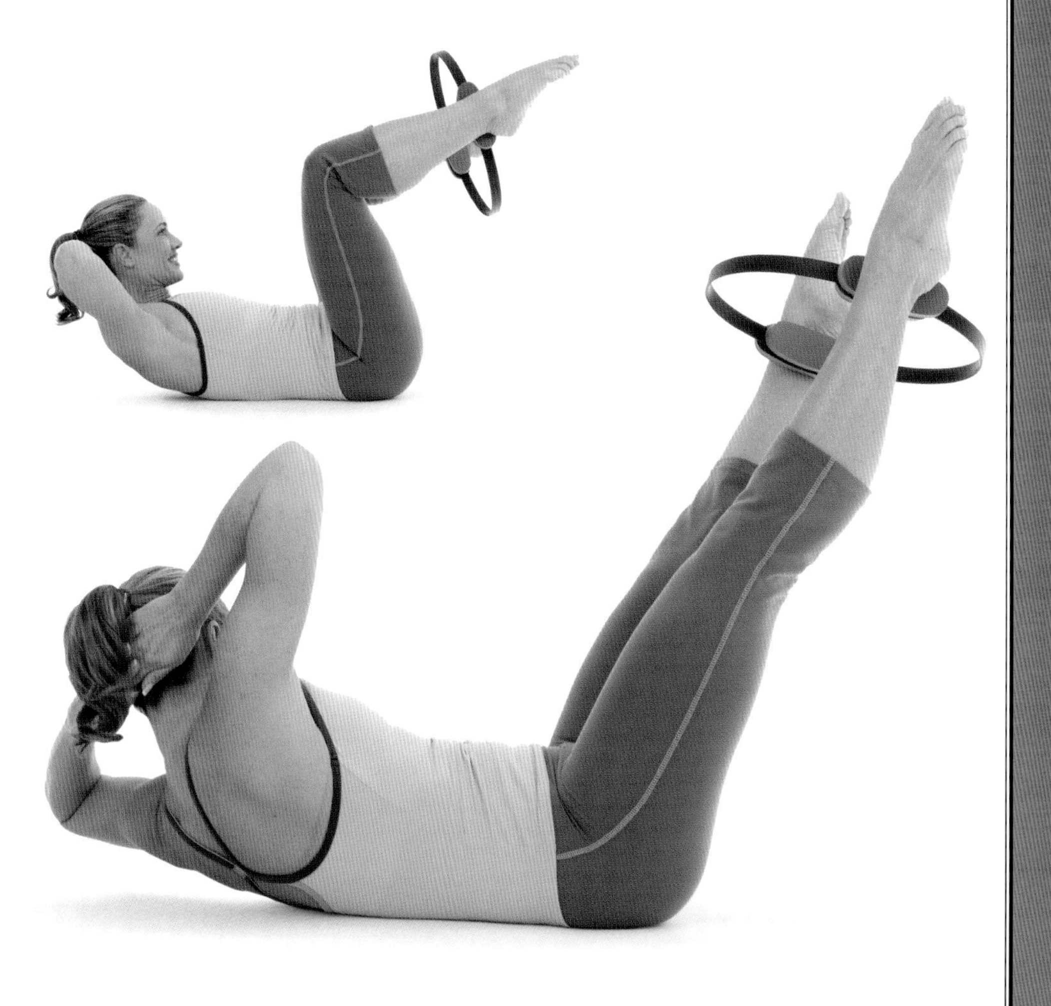

Spine Stretch Forward

Expands the breath, and stretches the spine and hamstrings.

1 Roll up off the mat and place your legs shoulder-width apart. Place the workout circle upright with one hand on top of the other.

2 Inhale. Squeeze your bottom; lift up off your bottom, keeping your chin on your chest. Exhale, scoop in and press down on the workout circle, drawing your powerhouse in deeper to fill out your lower back. Inhale to release the workout circle.

3 Repeat 2 times.

4 On the last one, place the workout circle aside, stretch your arms forward at shoulder level, chin to chest, and exhale as you peel down through your spine. Reach forward and then hold the arches of your feet. Inhale. As you exhale continue to pull the crown of your head down to the floor. Reach your arms forward and stack your vertebra one by one until you reach your tall, seated position.

Note

As you press the workout circle down, try to carve a deeper C-curve to fill out your lower back.

Relax your shoulders and make sure you are using your powerhouse to engage your workout circle.

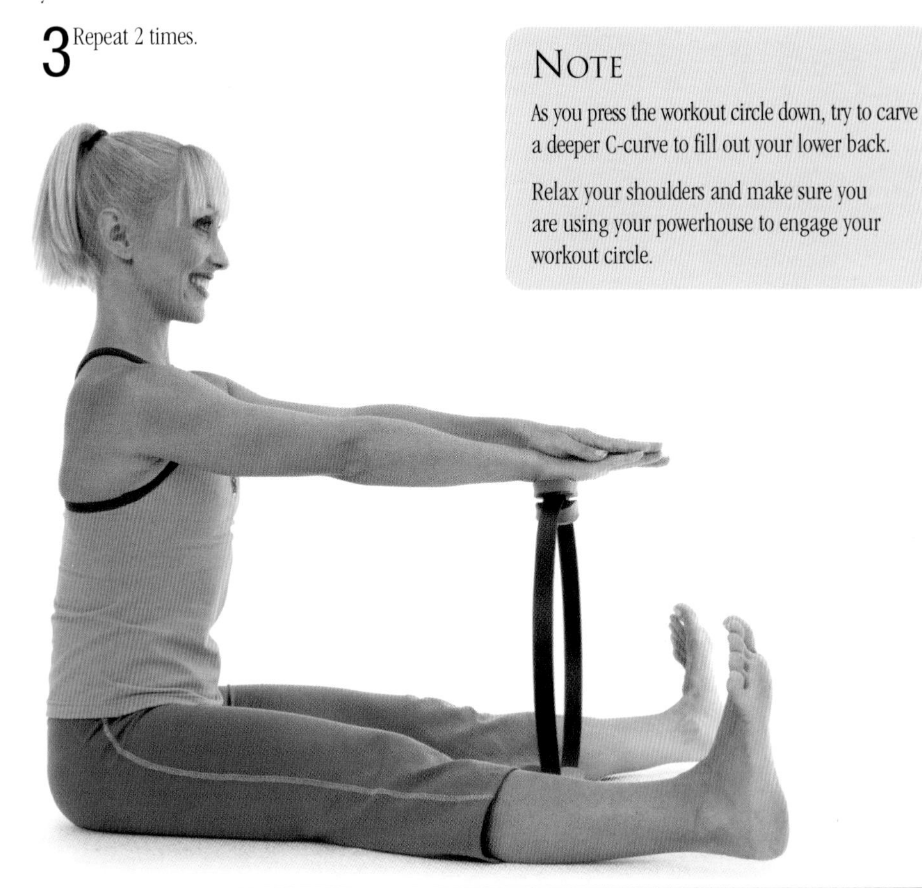

Modifications

Neck problems: Lower your gaze, rather than pressing your chin down to your chest.

Tight hamstrings: Bend your knees.

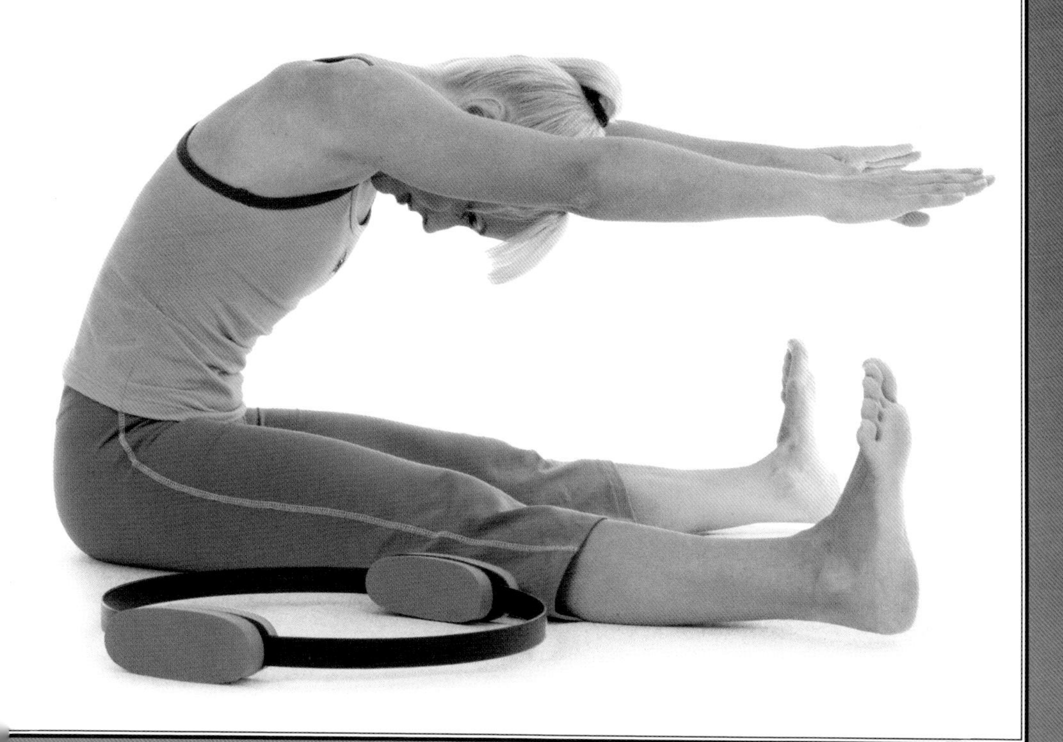

Open-Leg Rocker

Massages the spine and internal organs, and improves flexibility.

1 Sit forward at the edge of your mat and place the workout circle just above your ankles. Place your thumb and forefinger at the front of your ankle. Draw your heels into your bottom and balance while engaging the circle.

2 Extend your legs to shoulder-width and lift tall out of your lower back. Ensure you are squeezing your bottom and inner thighs to keep the workout circle engaged.

3 Inhale, drawing your chin to your chest. Exhale as you roll back and squeeze the workout circle, thinking of lifting your hips towards the ceiling. Inhale as you roll back up, lifting tall out of your spine, and balance.

4 Repeat 4 times.

Modifications

Lower back/disc problems: Complete only the balance; no rolling.

Tight hamstrings: Continue to do this exercise without the workout circle until your flexibility increases and you can straighten your legs.

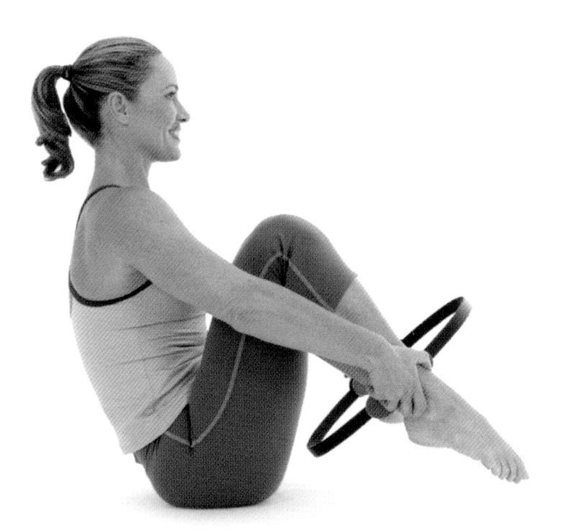

Note

Scoop in to initiate the roll backwards. Engage the workout circle from the bottom and inner thighs.

Do not initiate rolling backwards by swinging your head back and do not roll past your shoulder blades on to your neck. Do not sit into your lower back; keep lifted in your powerhouse.

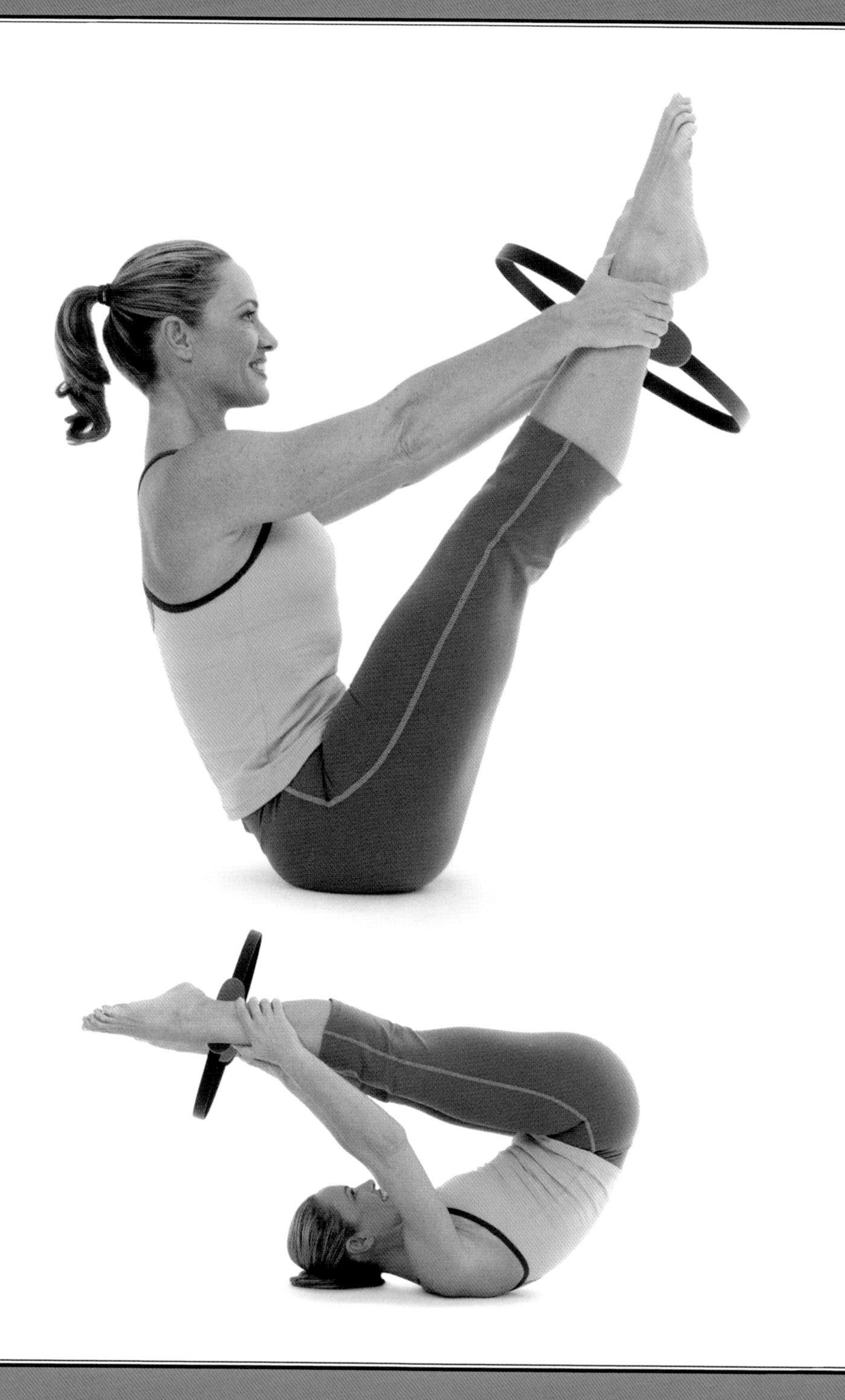

Corkscrew

Works the strength of the powerhouse and the sides of the body.

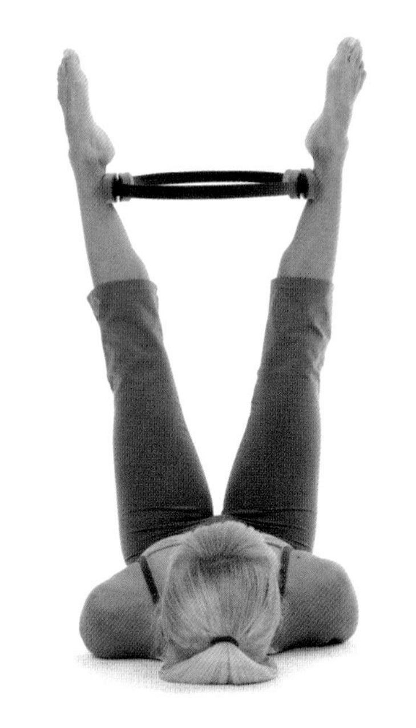

1 Scoop in and walk your hands down your legs, keeping the circle engaged. Lay down on the mat, hands by your sides with legs still extended towards the ceiling.

2 Keep the workout circle engaged with your bottom and inner thighs. Inhale. Draw a circle to the right and around to the left, and use your powerhouse to draw them back to the centre. Then draw your legs to the left around to the right and then back to the centre.

3 Intermediate level: Draw your legs to the right, around to the left and back to the centre. Squeezing your bottom and the workout circle, lift your hips, taking the first four vertebrae off the mat. Repeat towards the left side. Then repeat twice more, alternating sides.

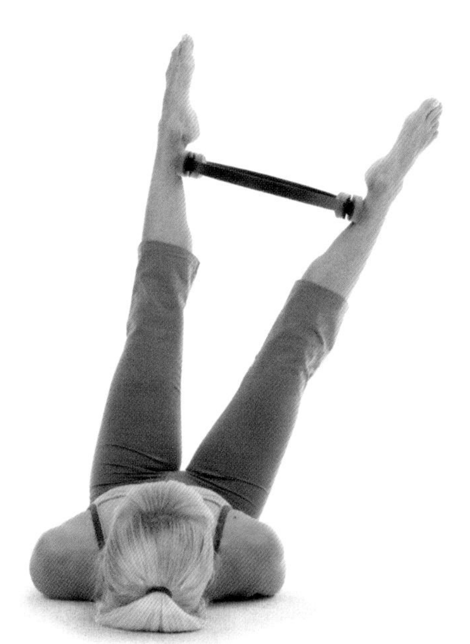

Note

Emphasise scooping your navel into your spine to keep your back flat. As your powerhouse gets stronger, draw a bigger circle.

Reduce the range of motion if you feel any back pain and omit the lift.

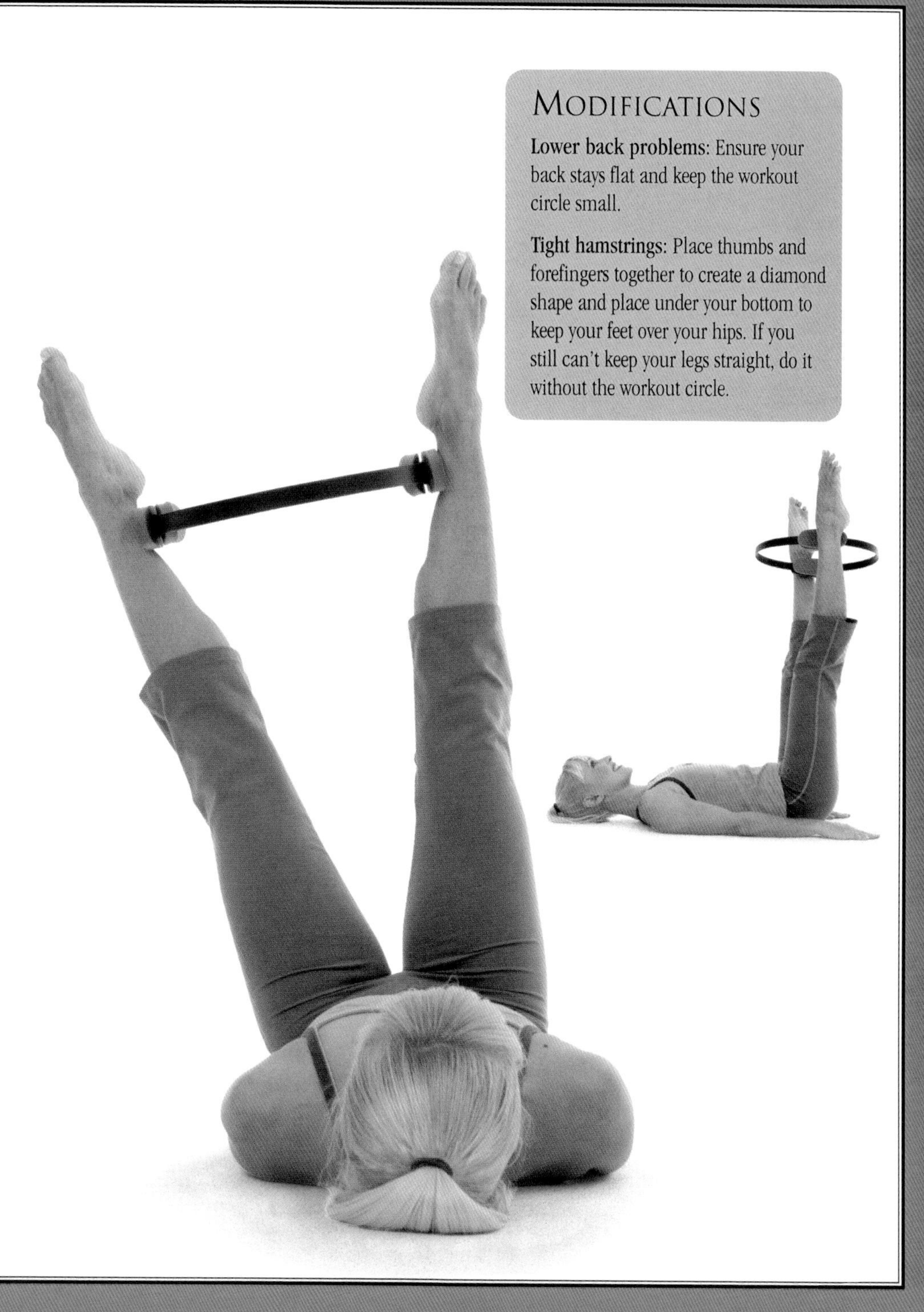

Modifications

Lower back problems: Ensure your back stays flat and keep the workout circle small.

Tight hamstrings: Place thumbs and forefingers together to create a diamond shape and place under your bottom to keep your feet over your hips. If you still can't keep your legs straight, do it without the workout circle.

The Saw

Eliminates stale air from the lungs, shapes the waistline and improves flexibility.

This exercise does not include the workout circle.

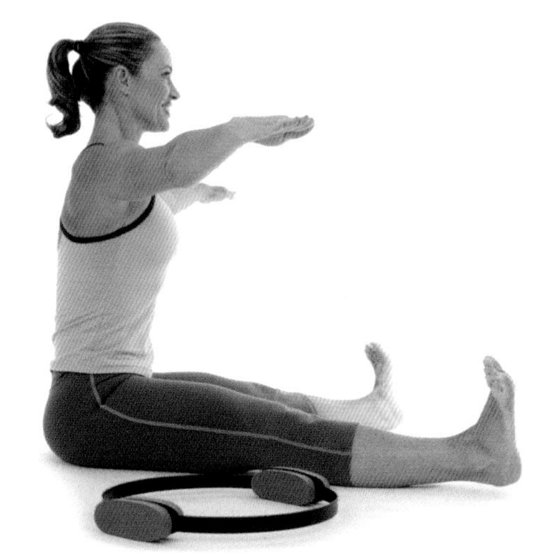

1 Sit up and open your legs, shoulder-width apart; flex your toes and reach through your heels. Reach your arms to the side, palms down (keeping arms in your peripheral vision).

2 Draw the powerhouse in and up. Inhale as you twist to the right from your stomach, working your waistline and lowering your back arm to protect your shoulder.

3 Exhale as you roll down through your spine, as you 'saw off' your little toe with your little finger. Keep both hips anchored to the mat. Scoop in and roll up through your spine and return to the centre.

4 Inhale and repeat to your left side.

5 Repeat 2 times each side.

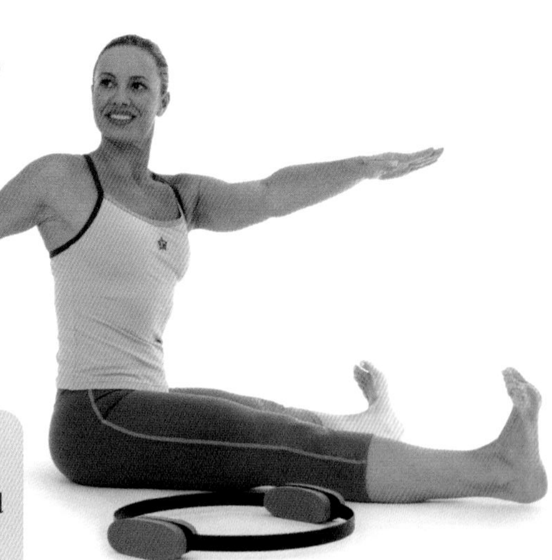

Note

Make sure you twist from your powerhouse and your waist, and not your shoulders or arms.

On the twist, try not to lift the hip you are twisting away from.

Modifications

Neck/back/disc problems: Omit this exercise.

Tight hamstrings: Keep knees soft.

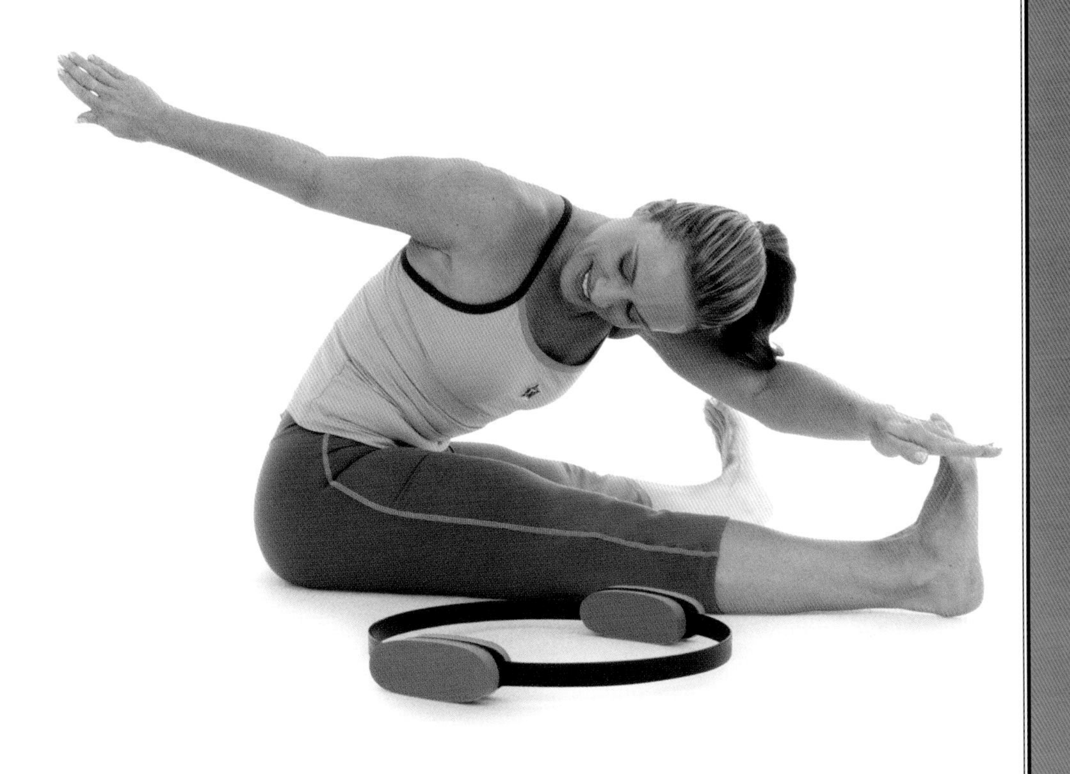

Prone Stomach Series

The next two exercises do not include the workout circle.

If any of these three exercises hurts your back, leave them out. Instead, continue working on strengthening your powerhouse, and then add them back in when you can.

Neck Roll

Stretches the neck and torso; supports the powerhouse and introduces spine extension.

1 Lie on your stomach with your feet together, hands in line with your ears and palms down. Scoop your stomach off the mat.

2 Inhale. Press into the palms of your hands, lifting your head and chest until you are either on your elbows or fully extended through your arms. Draw your shoulders down into your back, at the same time trying to keep your legs together. (When drawing up through the powerhouse, you should not feel it in your lower back.)

3 Inhale. Turn your head to the right, stretching your neck. Roll your head down across your chest and to the left and return to the centre. Look to the left, roll your head down across your chest and to the right. Look to the centre. Lift in your powerhouse, exhale, and lower yourself back down on to the mat.

4 Repeat once, alternating the neck roll left to right.

Note

Keep your powerhouse lifted off the mat and work with your legs together.

If you feel any lower back pain, reduce the range of motion – come up only to your elbows.

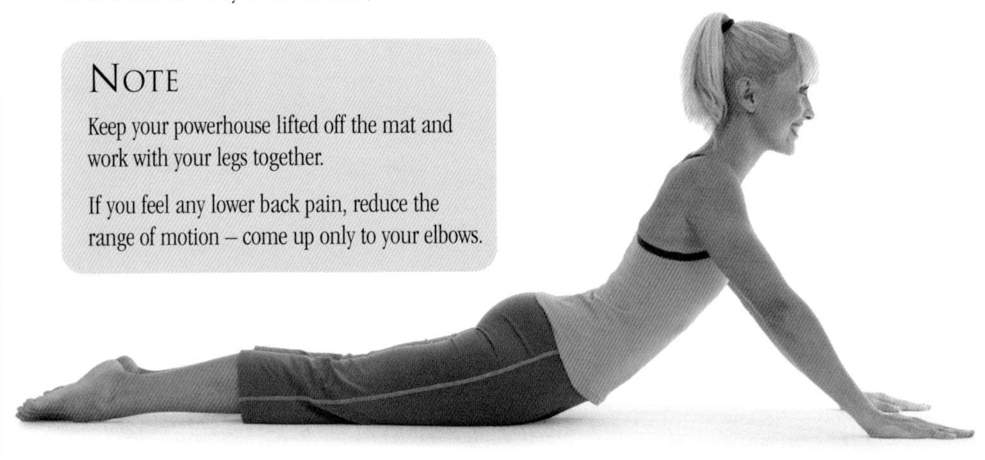

Modifications

Lower back/disc problems: Omit this exercise.

Neck/elbow/shoulder problems: Omit this exercise.

Weak neck: Do not roll your head.

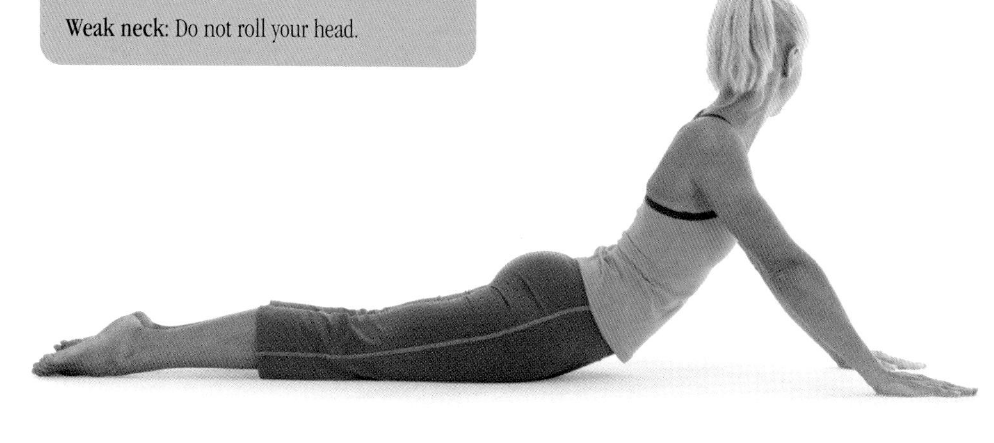

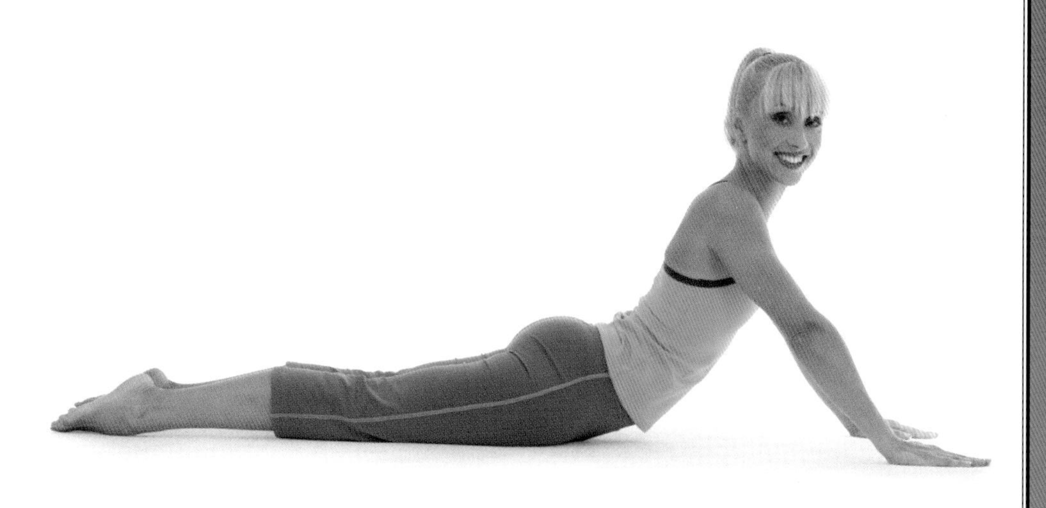

SINGLE-LEG KICKS

Stretches the front of the body and the quadriceps

1 Once you finish your last neck roll, come up on to your elbows, fists pressed firmly into the floor (sphinx position). Draw your shoulders down into your back, draw the stomach and ribcage off the mat, lift your chest and keep your chin up.

2 Try to keep your knees together. Kick your right leg with double pulse to your bottom while keeping your other leg extended on the mat. Switch legs and pulse opposite heel to your bottom. Try not to sink into your lower back. Keep your powerhouse scooped in so your stomach is off the mat and your chest is lifted towards the ceiling.

3 Repeat 4 times.

NOTE

Keep looking ahead and scoop your powerhouse in as you kick your heel to your bottom.

Try to keep your knees together as you kick your heel to your bottom and do not sink into your shoulders or lower back.

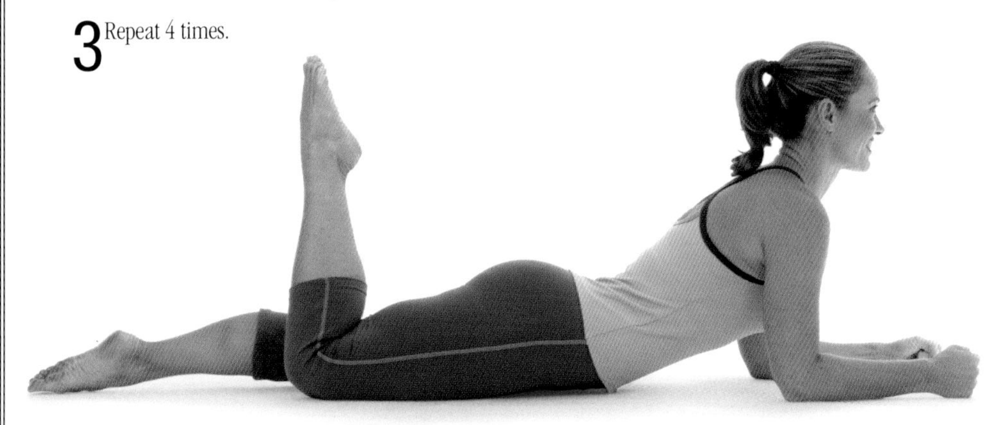

MODIFICATIONS

Lower back /disc problems: Omit this exercise.

Elbow/shoulder/knee problems: Omit this exercise.

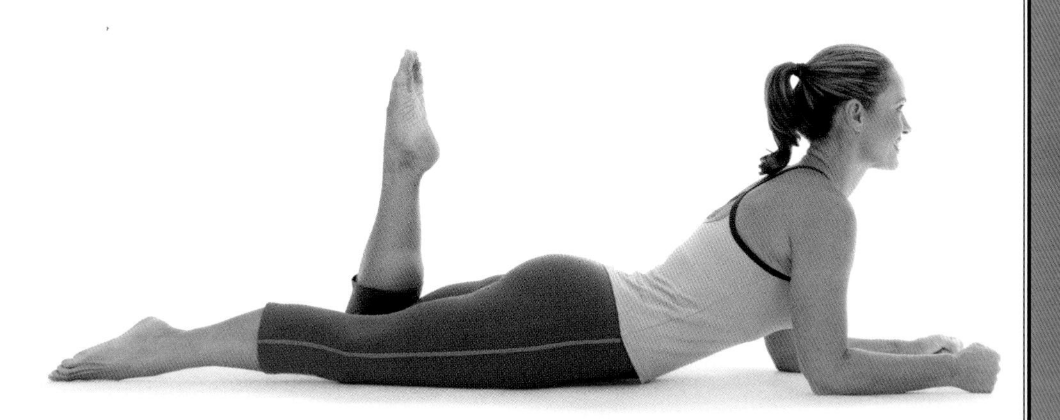

DOUBLE-LEG KICKS

Stretches the upper back and shoulders and opens the chest.

1 Continuing to lie face down on the mat, hold the workout circle between your hands, place your right cheek on the mat and place the workout circle as high up on to your shoulders as possible, allowing your elbows to touch the mat.

2 Draw your navel into your spine. Inhale. Kick both heels to your bottom three times and return your legs long to the mat. Exhaling, lift your head and chest up off the mat. Stretch your arms and squeeze the workout circle with the heels of your hands. Still holding the workout circle, reach down to the back of your thighs, squeezing your shoulder-blades together and opening your chest. Try to keep your toes on the mat.

3 Return to the mat, place your left cheek down and keep your hands as high up on your back as possible.

4 Repeat 3 times.

MODIFICATIONS

Lower back/disc problems: Omit this exercise.

Elbow/neck/shoulder/knee problems: Omit this exercise.

NOTE

Try to lengthen your spine as you extend and lift off the mat.

Keep the kick small to minimise movement through your torso.

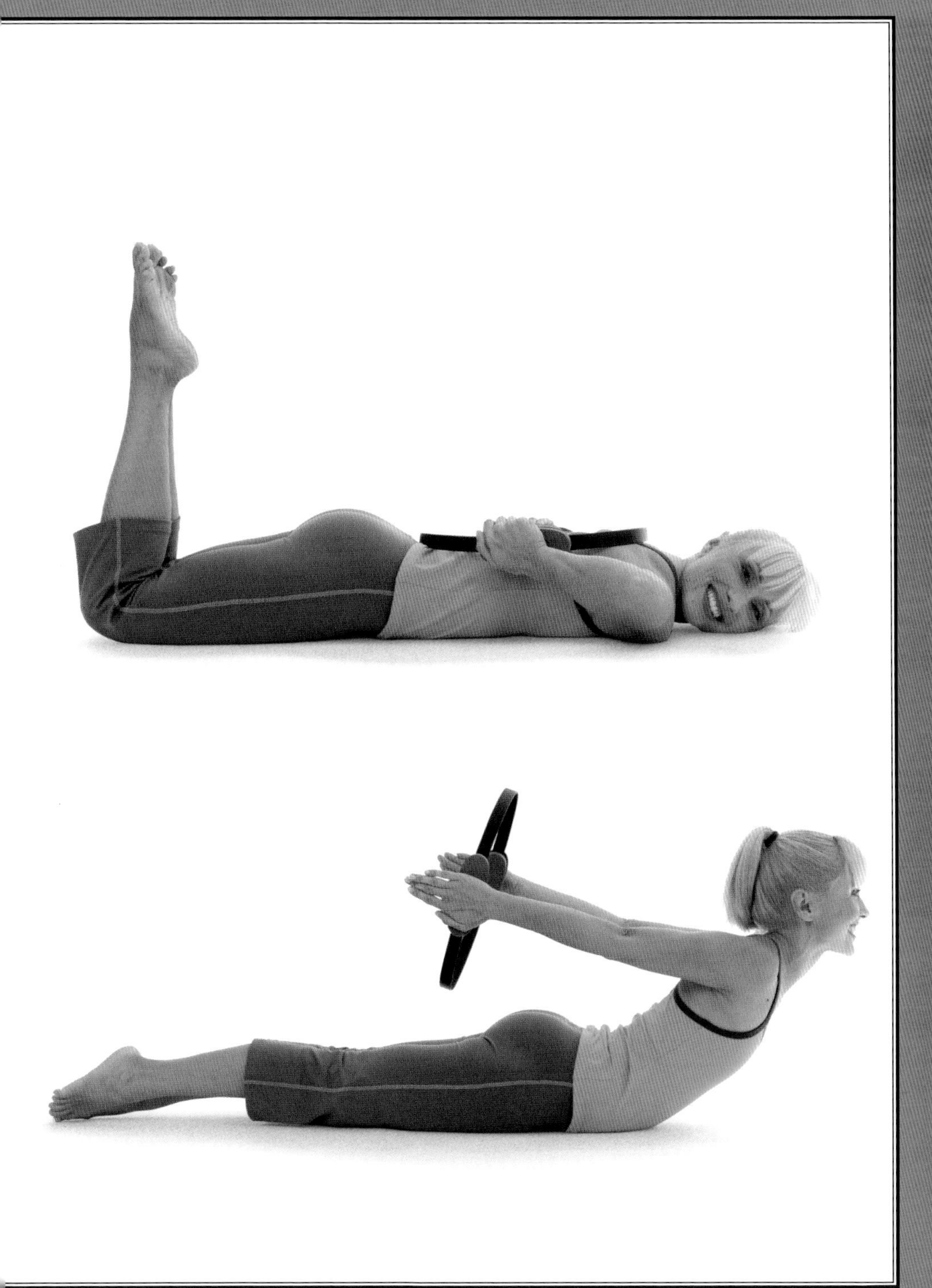

Neck Pull

Works the powerhouse, stretches the hamstrings, and lengthens and articulates the spine.

1 Lie flat on your back with your legs extended hip-width apart. Place the workout circle flat on the floor and flex your toes and hold the workout circle with your heels. Place your hands behind your head, one on top of the other.

2 Inhale. Scoop in and draw your chin to your chest engaging the workout circle from your bottom and inner thighs. Roll up off the mat.

3 Exhale. Scoop in deeper and round over (as if over a big beach ball). Keep your heels flexed and off the floor.

4 Inhale. Roll up, stacking your spine vertebra by vertebra. Keep your spine lengthened and squeeze your bottom and the workout circle. Draw your navel in to your spine and peel down on to the mat, lengthening your spine as you reach out through your heels.

5 Repeat 4 times.

Note

As you roll up, really reach through your heels squeezing your bottom and inner thighs.

If your feet are lifting while rolling up, stretch your arms forward to the side of your thighs and lightly walk up using your fingertips, maintaining the C-curve at all times.

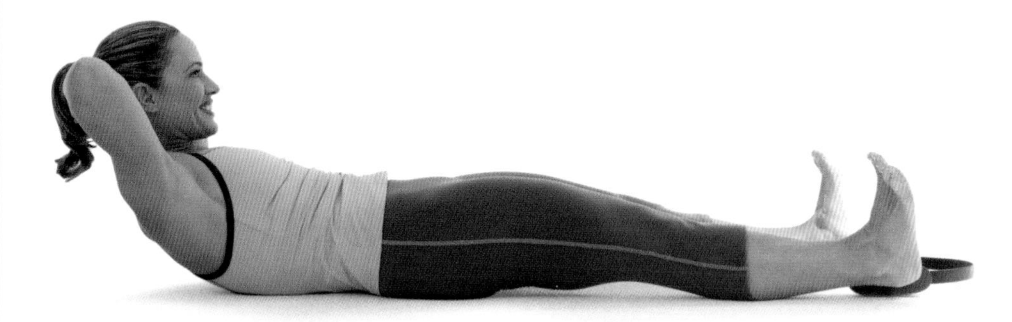

Modifications

Weak/lower back problems: Omit the workout circle. Bend your knees and use your hands to walk up and down your legs during the rolling sequences.

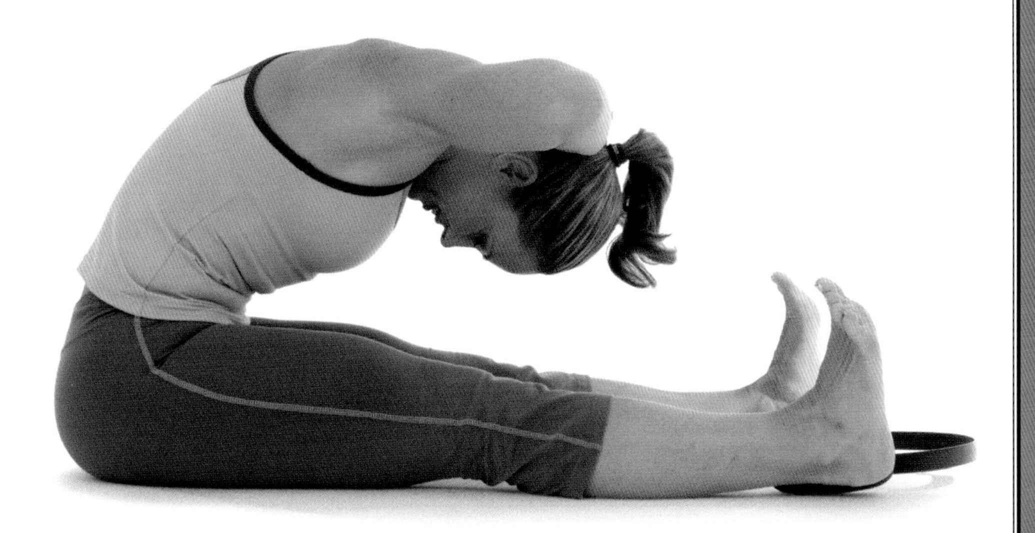

Side-Kick Series

The following series works inner and outer thighs, strengthens glutes and increases flexibility; excellent for finding balance and symmetry.

The next three exercises do not include the workout circle.

Both this series and the following Lying-Leg series are to be completed on one side first and then, after the Transition, they are repeated on the other side.

Forward/Back

1 Lie on your side, on the back edge of your mat, your elbow in line with your hips, hips in line with your feet. Bring your feet forward to a 45-degree angle. Place your other hand behind your head. Keep the rib cage closed.

2 Lengthen your top leg out of your hip socket so that your heels are one on top of the other. Lift your leg to hip height and, keeping your hips stacked, rotate your leg from your hip so your knee faces the ceiling.

3 Using your powerhouse, kick your leg forward with a double-pulse movement. Without moving your torso, reach down and back as you stretch your leg behind you.

4 Repeat 7 times.

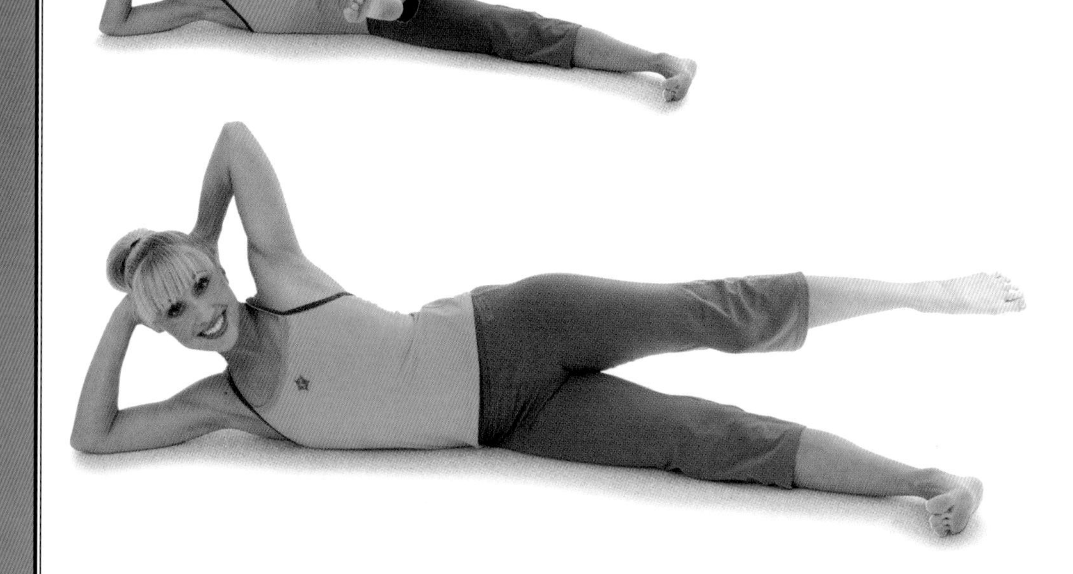

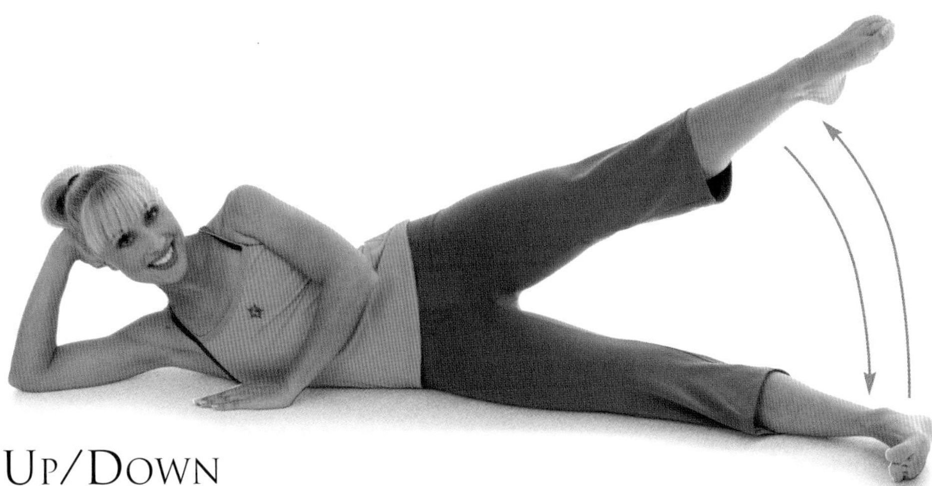

Up/Down

1 Maintaining the same position as the previous exercise, place your hand back on the mat and bring your heels together. Lift one leg and slightly rotate it so your knee points to the ceiling. Stretch your leg long out of your hip.

2 Make sure your hip doesn't roll back behind you. (Your hips should always stay stacked as you lift your leg.) Lower, resisting on the way down as if you are trying to burst a balloon between your inner thighs.

3 Repeat 4 times and then bring your heels together.

Small Circles

1 In the same position, lift your top leg to hip height, keeping your shoulders and hips stacked. Rotate your leg in small circles in one direction five times and then repeat in the opposite direction.

2 Aim to brush your heels together and squeeze your inner thighs as they touch while you are making the circles.

3 Make sure you keep your legs one on top of the other during this exercise.

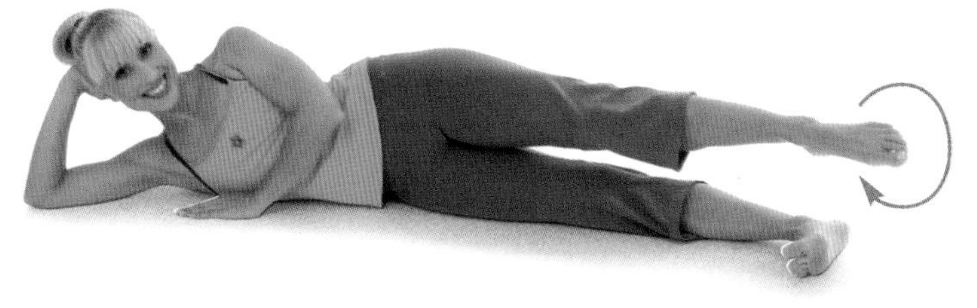

Lying-Leg Series

To tone outer and inner thighs, and strengthen the powerhouse.

Press Down

1 Maintain the same position as the previous series. Take the workout circle and place it between your legs. Your underneath leg should be placed through the workout circle, pressing down on the bottom pad. Your top leg should be placed on the top pad.

2 Slightly rotate your top leg from your bottom and inner thighs. Keep a soft knee and press down and hold for 3 counts (visualise trying to burst a balloon between your thighs).

3 Repeat 2 times.

4 Keep your movements small and controlled. Press down and pulse for 3 counts.

5 Repeat 3 times.

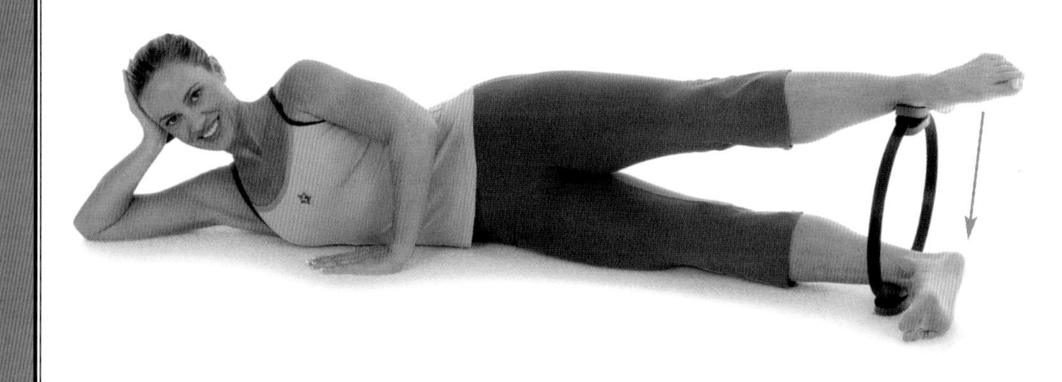

Press Up

1 Place your top leg through the workout circle so the outside of your leg is pressing up against the pad. Press up and hold for 3 counts.

2 Repeat 2 times. Add 3 small pulses. Repeat 3 times.

3 Carefully move your top leg back on to the outside of the workout circle, roll the workout circle backwards and place your underneath leg on the outside of the bottom pad.

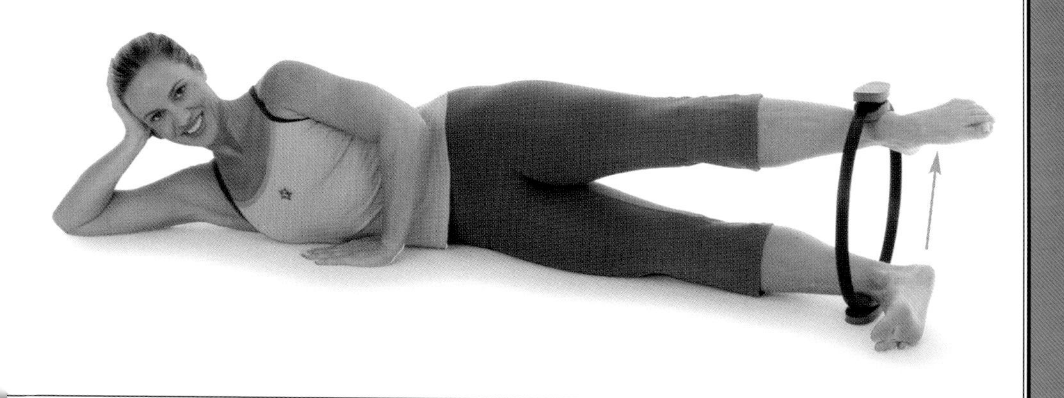

LEG LIFTS

Roll back on to your side so your hips and shoulders are stacked. Squeezing your bottom and inner thighs, raise both legs off the mat, engaging the workout circle, and pulse for 10 counts, maintaining the lift through your powerhouse at all times.

NOTE

Try to keep your torso stable, long and lengthened throughout these exercises. Remember to keep your hips stacked one on top of the other.

Remember not to emphasise the squeeze of the workout circle with your knees. Use your bottom and inner thighs.

MODIFICATIONS

These modifications apply to all exercises in the Side-Kick and Lying-Leg series.

Lower back/sciatic nerve problems: Keep range of motion smaller. If suffering sciatic pain, omit the Up/Down and the Lying-Leg series.

Elbow/wrist/shoulder/neck problems: Lay flat with a long arm, head on a small pillow.

For men (with tighter hips): Only do side-kicks forward and back.

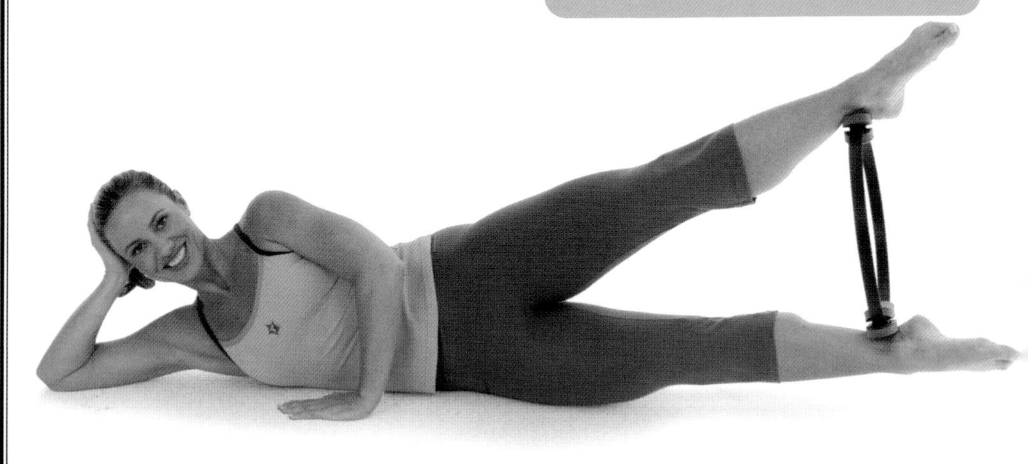

TRANSITION

1 Keeping the workout circle engaged, roll on to your stomach, and place one hand on top of the other on the mat. Place your forehead into your hands.

2 Squeeze the workout circle from your bottom and inner thighs, scoop your powerhouse in and lift your legs off the mat. Pulse the workout circle 20 times.

3 Roll over to repeat the Side-Kick series and the Lying-Leg series on your other side.

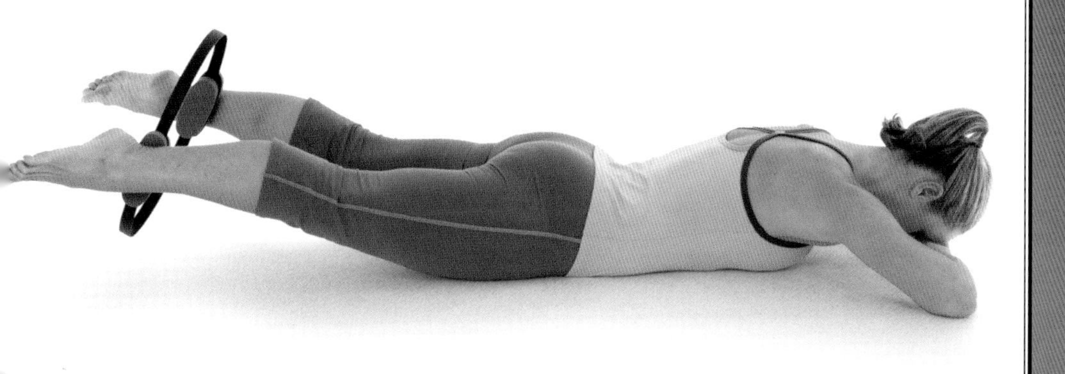

Teaser

Improves balance and control, and strengthens the powerhouse.

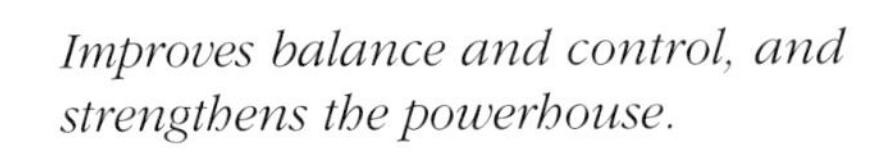

Teaser Preparation 1

1 Lie on your back, with your knees bent and together. Squeeze your bottom and inner thighs. Holding the workout circle in your hands, bring your arms over your head so your back is flat and your ribs are closed. Draw your navel towards your spine.

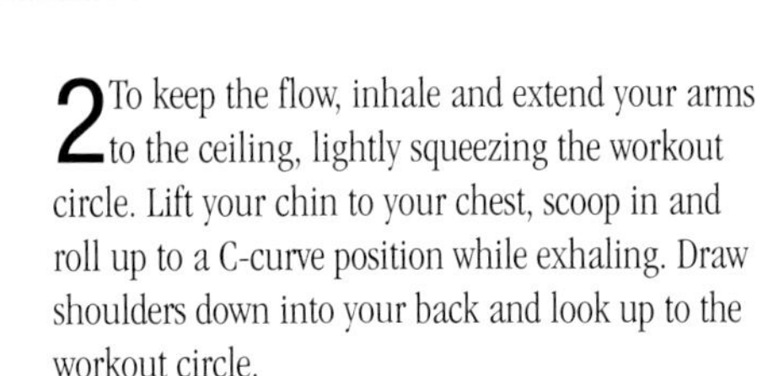

2 To keep the flow, inhale and extend your arms to the ceiling, lightly squeezing the workout circle. Lift your chin to your chest, scoop in and roll up to a C-curve position while exhaling. Draw shoulders down into your back and look up to the workout circle.

3 Inhale. With your chin to your chest, scoop in deeper and peel your spine down to the mat, pressing your feet into the floor and squeezing your inner thighs and bottom.

4 As you roll down, make sure your head touches the mat first. Exhale and extend your arms back behind your head.

5 Repeat 2 times.

Teaser Preparation 2

1 Lie on your back with your knees bent and together. Extend your right leg, squeezing your inner thighs (do not let your leg rest on your other knee), and extend your arms over your head as you hold the workout circle.

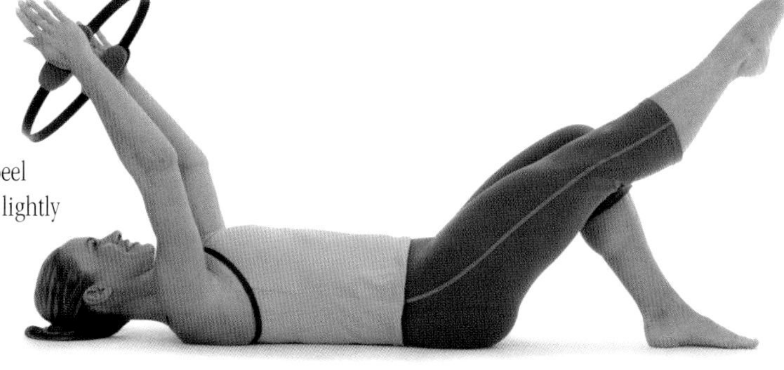

2 Inhale. Bring your arms forward, chin to your chest, and, while exhaling, peel your spine off the mat while lightly squeezing the workout circle to engage your powerhouse (keep squeezing your thighs together). Holding the workout circle, reach towards the extended toe.

3 With your chin to your chest roll back down to the mat maintaining the squeeze through your bottom and inner thighs. Draw your shoulders down and exhale as you bring your arms back over your head.

4 Repeat with your left leg extended.

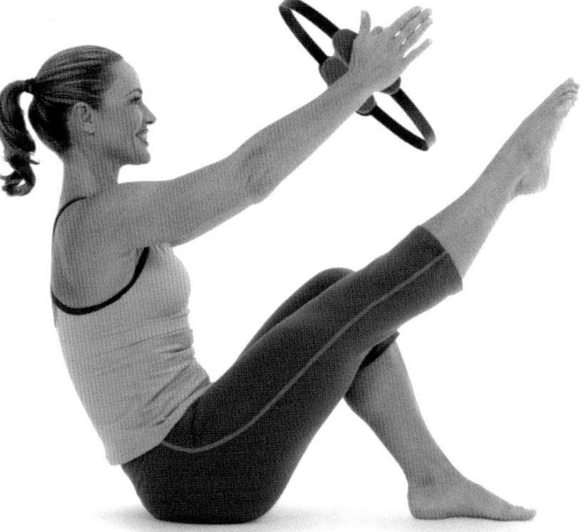

Modifications

Lower back problems: Omit the workout circle. As you inhale, bring your arms forward, chin to your chest, scoop in, peel up off the mat and walk your hands up your legs.

TEASER

You should master Teaser Preparations 1 and 2 before moving on to this exercise.

1 Lie on your back and place the workout circle between your ankles. Bring your knees to your chest and extend your arms over your head, keeping your ribs closed. Scoop your powerhouse in, extend your legs to a 45-degree angle, ensuring you are engaging the workout circle through your bottom and inner thighs and that your back stays flat on the mat.

2 Bring your arms forward, chin to your chest. Inhale, scoop in and roll up through your powerhouse to the Teaser position. Exhale as you reach your fingertips to your toes.

3 Inhale, chin to your chest. Draw your powerhouse in and peel your spine back down on to the mat, leaving your legs at a 45-degree angle, circle engaged.

4 Repeat twice, finishing by drawing your knees into your chest.

NOTE

Make sure you keep your legs at a 45-degree angle, engaging your glutes and inner thighs to hold the workout circle in place.

If you find your back is arching off the mat, stay with Teaser Preparations 1 and 2 until you are stronger.

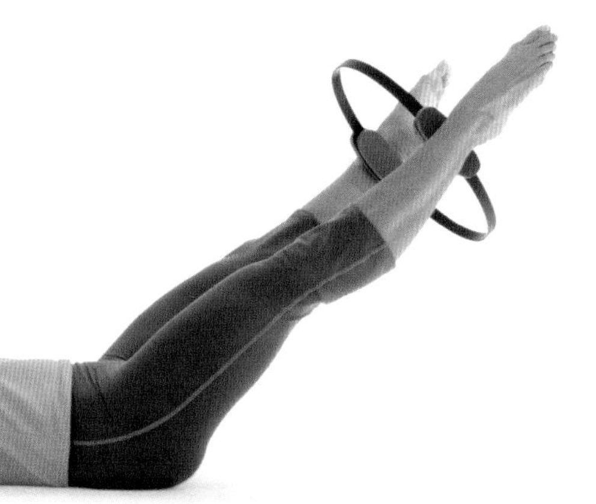

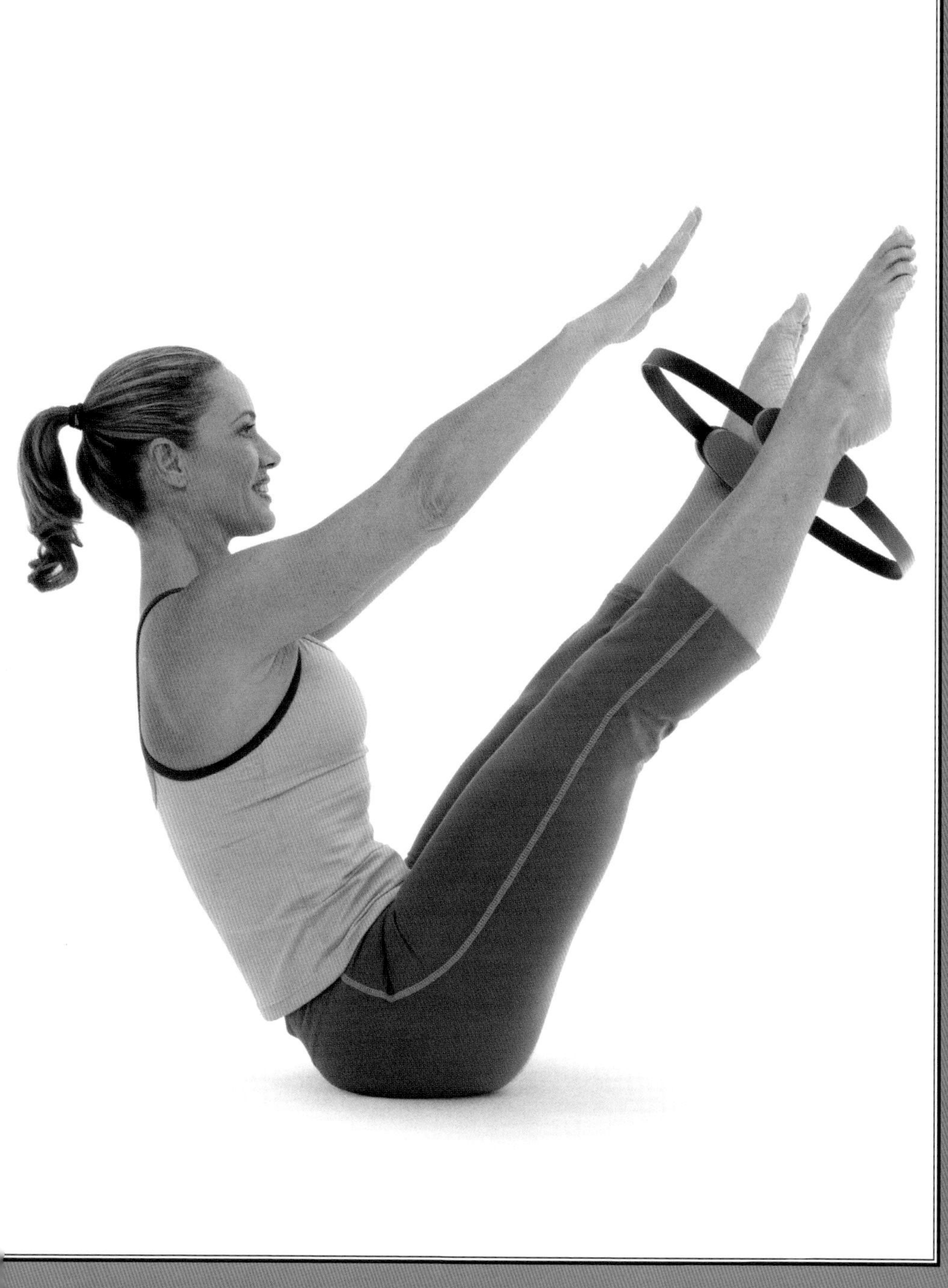

The Seal

An exercise to massage the spine, work the powerhouse, and improve balance and control.

This exercise does not include the workout circle.

1 Sit at the end of the mat. Bring the soles of your feet together; separate your knees so they are shoulder-width apart. Place your hands inside your legs and grasp the outside of your feet.

2 Draw your navel into your spine and your chin to your chest. As you lift your feet off the mat and balance, carve a deep C-curve with your torso. Clap your feet together three times by squeezing your inner thighs, inhale and initiate rolling back from your powerhouse.

3 Roll only on to your shoulder blades, and not on your neck. Control your roll and clap your feet together three times over your head. Scoop in deeper, exhale and roll back up.

4 Hold your balance on your sitting bones at the end of each roll, scooping in.

5 Repeat 4 times. On the last roll, let go of your legs as you roll back up and stand on the mat in the Pilates stance, ready for the Push-Ups.

Modifications

Back/neck problems: Omit this exercise.

Shoulder/elbow problems: Omit this exercise.

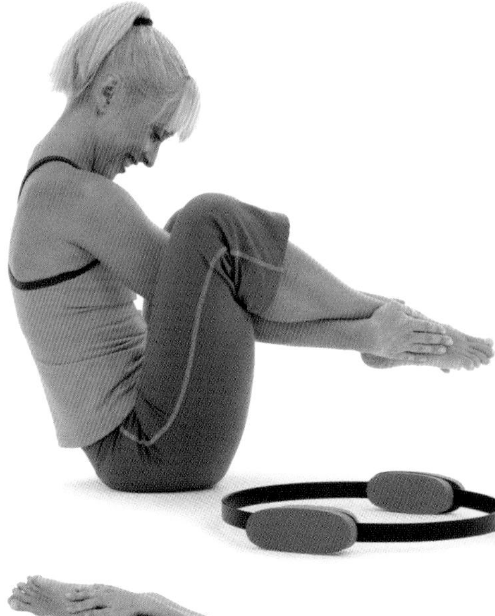

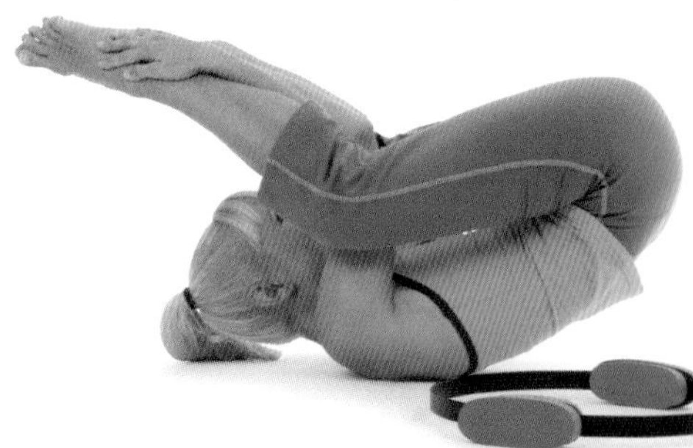

Note

Enjoy the massage on your spine.

Try not to initiate the roll by throwing your head back. Make sure you control the rolling and do not roll on to your neck.

PUSH-UPS

Works the upper body, strengthens the powerhouse and increases flexibility.

This exercise does not include the workout circle.

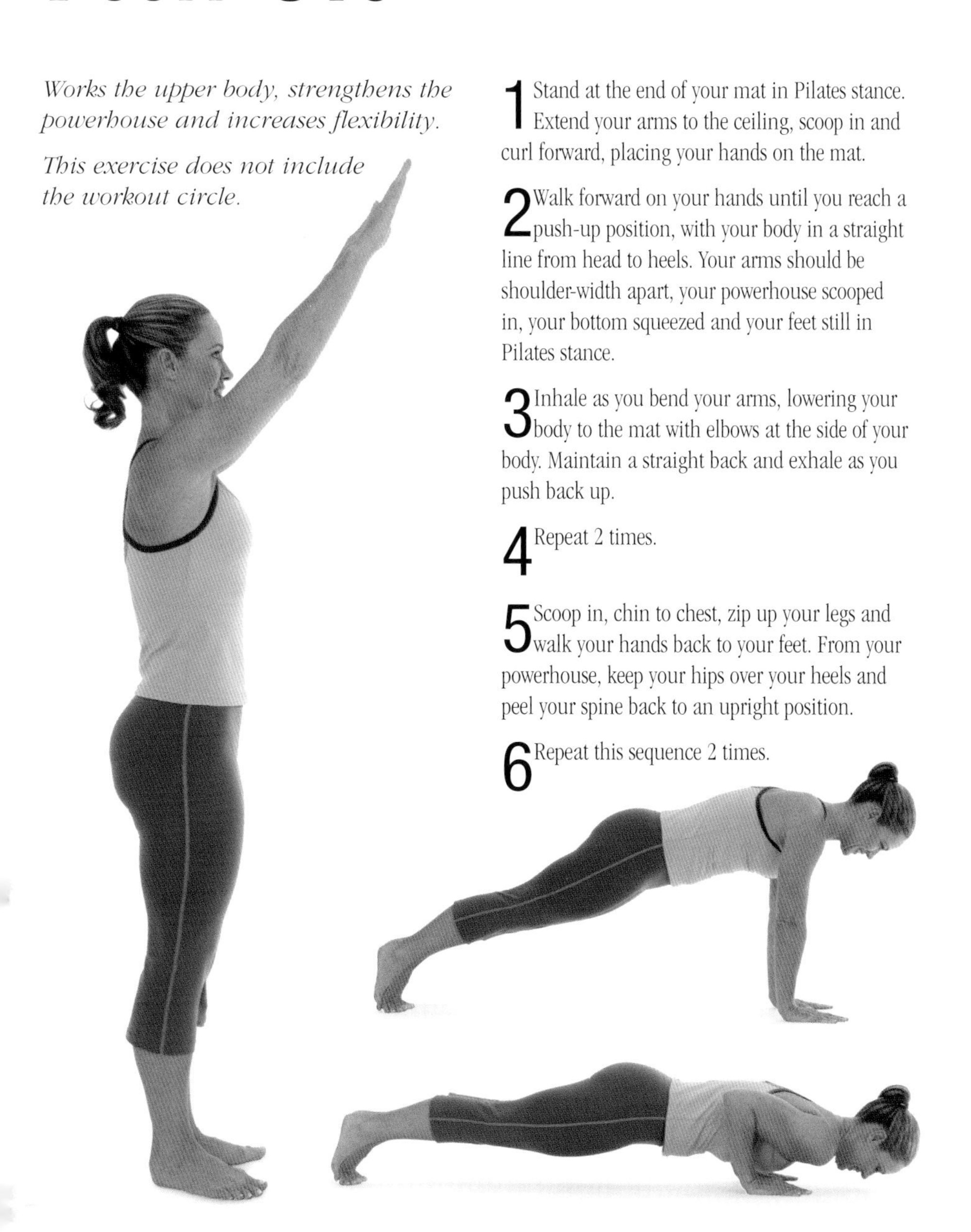

1 Stand at the end of your mat in Pilates stance. Extend your arms to the ceiling, scoop in and curl forward, placing your hands on the mat.

2 Walk forward on your hands until you reach a push-up position, with your body in a straight line from head to heels. Your arms should be shoulder-width apart, your powerhouse scooped in, your bottom squeezed and your feet still in Pilates stance.

3 Inhale as you bend your arms, lowering your body to the mat with elbows at the side of your body. Maintain a straight back and exhale as you push back up.

4 Repeat 2 times.

5 Scoop in, chin to chest, zip up your legs and walk your hands back to your feet. From your powerhouse, keep your hips over your heels and peel your spine back to an upright position.

6 Repeat this sequence 2 times.

STANDING ARM SERIES

The workout circle is used predominantly to strengthen the upper body and tone and shape the arms. It is also beneficial for postural awareness, to help lift from the arches (while standing), for engaging the powerhouse and maintaining a balanced, centred position while working the upper body.

Begin this series by taking up the Pilates stance. Make sure you are not rolling in your ankles or arches. Keep your weight on your toes. Zip up your inner thighs, squeeze your bottom, pull your navel in and up, close your rib cage, open across your chest and collarbone and draw your shoulders down into your back.

Each time you squeeze or pulse the workout circle, try to get a deeper connection with your powerhouse rather than just using the strength of your upper body. Remember to keep the fingers long and relaxed, adding pressure to the workout circle from the heel of the hands. Remember, the workout circle works with the powerhouse.

CHEST

1 In Pilates stance, keep your weight forward over your toes, hold the workout circle with the heels of your hands and lift the workout circle to chest level.

2 Draw your shoulders down into your back and keep your rib cage closed. Squeeze the workout circle from your chest muscles and hold for 3 counts. Try not to shorten your arms as you do this but keep the elbows lifted.

3 Release and repeat twice.

4 Engaging the workout circle, add 3 small pulses and release.

5 Repeat twice.

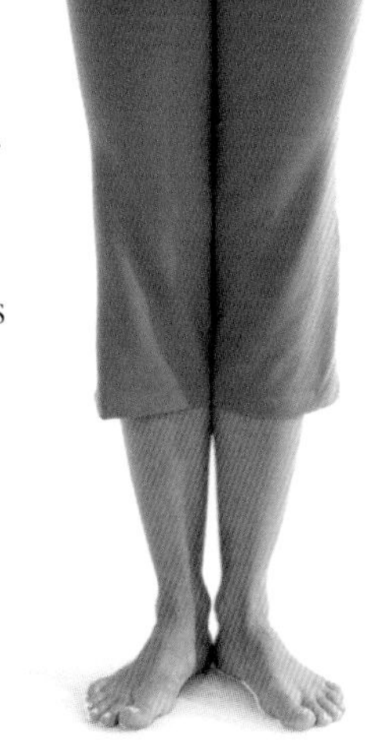

Hip

1 Lower the workout circle to hip level, keeping your elbows soft and arms long. Make sure your shoulders are relaxed and pulled down into your back.

2 Squeeze the workout circle once again, repeating the sequence of the squeeze. Hold for the count of 3 and repeat 3 times.

3 Repeat the small pulses 3 times.

Head

1 Extend your arms forward and up to create the effect of a halo, keeping the weight forward over your toes.

2 Draw your shoulders down, close your rib cage. Scoop in and repeat the sequence of the squeeze and hold. Repeat 3 times.

Up/Down

1 Take the workout circle back to hip level.

2 Using the last three positions, pulse the workout circle 8–10 times by moving up your body, starting from hip level to chest level and then head level. Hold at the top, pull your shoulders down, scoop in and pulse down 8–10 times back to hip level. Try not to shorten your arms throughout this sequence.

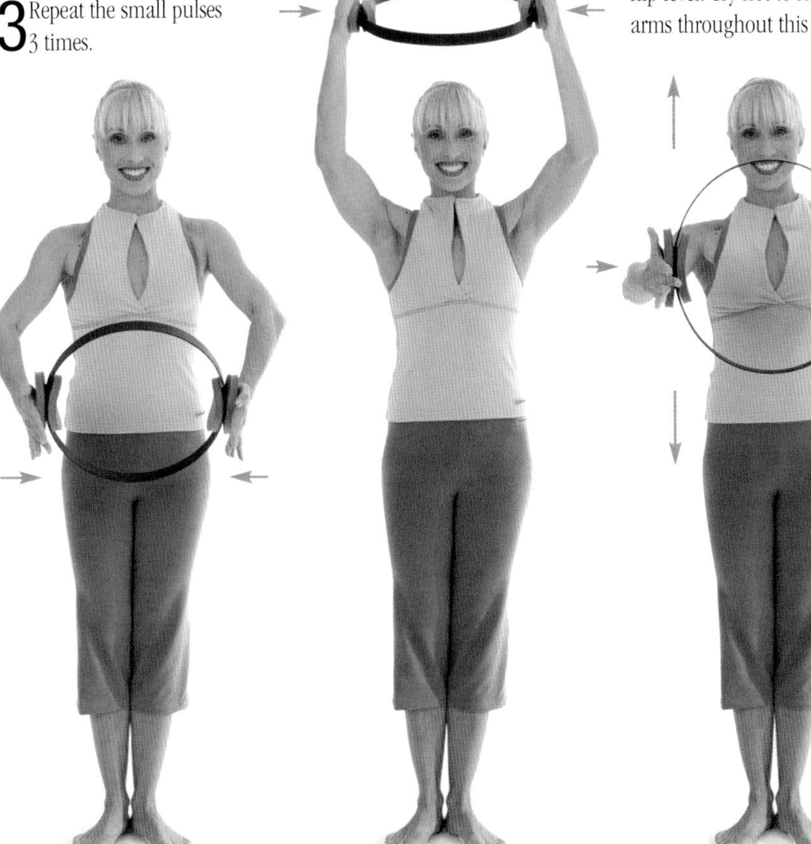

Standing Arm Series *(continued)*

Back

1 Take the workout circle behind your lower back (still in the heels of your hands). Draw your shoulders down, close your rib cage, scoop in and try to engage the workout circle. (Do not worry if you can't squeeze the workout circle. Just initiating the movement is a workout in itself.)

2 Hold for the count of 6.

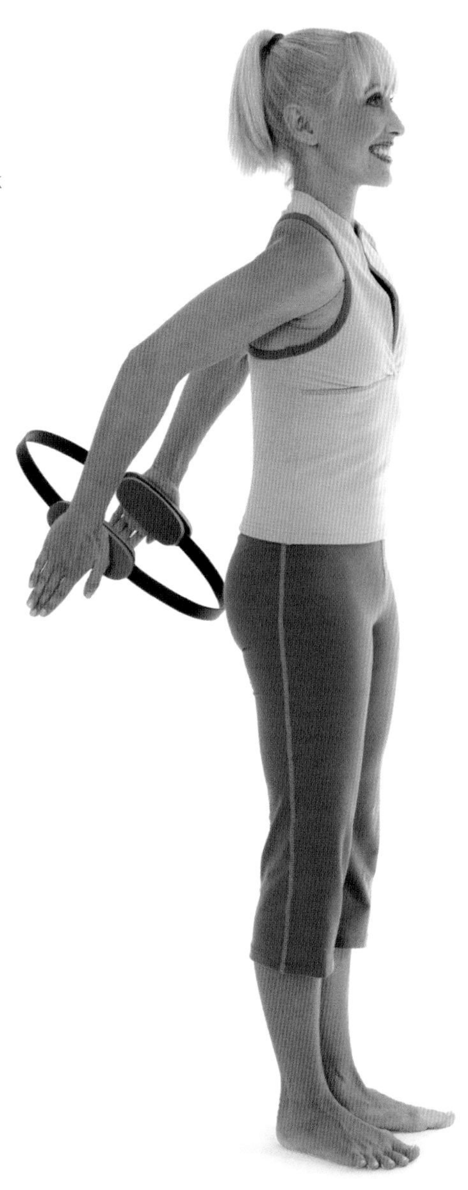

Side-Arm

1 Place the workout circle just below your hip bone, with your other hand by your side.

2 Lift your elbow up, and try to draw your shoulder down into your back.

3 Squeeze the workout circle in towards your body using your back – and not your shoulder or elbow – without shortening your arm. Release and repeat twice more.

4 Pulse 3 small pulses and then reverse sides. Repeat twice.

5 Change sides and repeat the exercise.

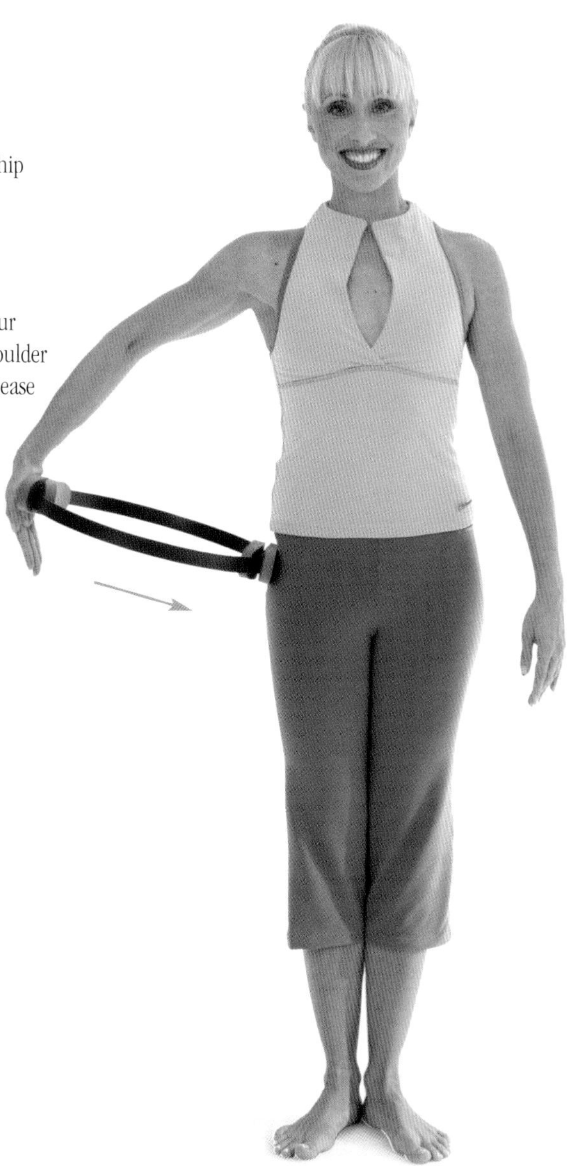

STANDING LEG SEQUENCE

Ideal for shaping the bottom and thighs.

Begin this sequence by placing the workout circle just above your ankles. The workout circle should stay in this position throughout the leg sequence. It is important to maintain correct posture. (Start this sequence holding on to the back of a chair until you can balance alone.) Keep pulling your powerhouse in to stay lengthened from the top of your head.

FRONT/SIDE

1 In the Pilates stance, hold the workout circle between your legs, just above your ankles. Extend your arms out to the side. Scoop in, as if you are being pulled through the crown of your head. Transfer your weight on to your right leg and lift your left leg into the air, engaging your bottom and wrapping your thighs. Make sure you are pulling up on the standing leg.

2 Squeeze the workout circle by engaging your bottom and drawing your inner thighs together and then release. Repeat 9 times.

3 Scoop in deeper and then bring your left foot forward with the workout circle still between your ankles. Pull up through your torso, engaging your bottom and squeezing the workout circle as you visualise your legs drawing together. Repeat 9 times.

4 Bring your left leg back to your side, and then transfer your weight over so the right leg is now in the air. Keep scooping and lifting tall. Squeeze the workout circle together from your inner thighs and release. Repeat 9 times.

5 Bring your right leg forward and squeeze and release. Repeat 9 times. Bring your right leg back to the side and lower.

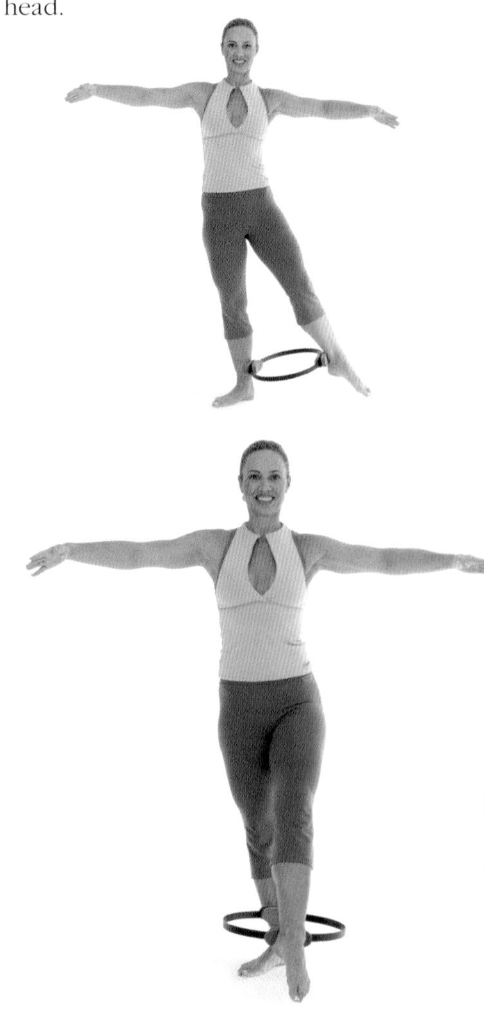

Seated Leg Sequence

Focuses on the bottom, and inner and outer thighs.

1 Sit on a chair, bed or sofa, so that your hips and knees are in line.

2 Place the workout circle just above your knees on your inner thighs.

3 Lift your arms and cross them at chest height. Lift up tall in your powerhouse and scoop in.

4 Squeeze your bottom, pull your stomach in deeper and squeeze the workout circle together using your inner thighs. Hold and try to change the shape of the circle.

5 Release and then repeat 5 times.

Mat Table

1

The Hundred
Inhale 5 counts
Exhale 5 counts
x 10

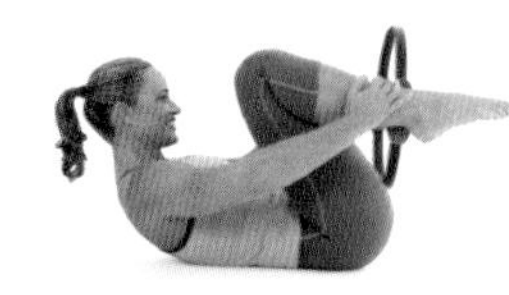

2

The Roll-Up
x 5

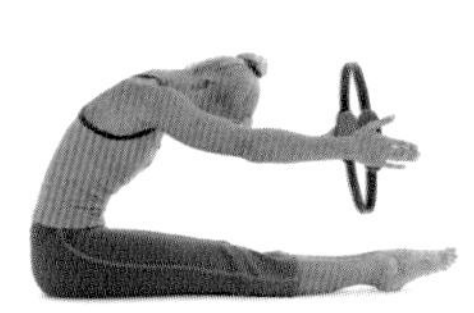

3

Single-Leg Circles
x 5 each way.
Repeat other leg.

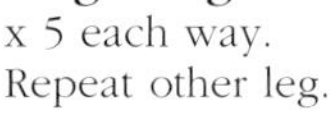

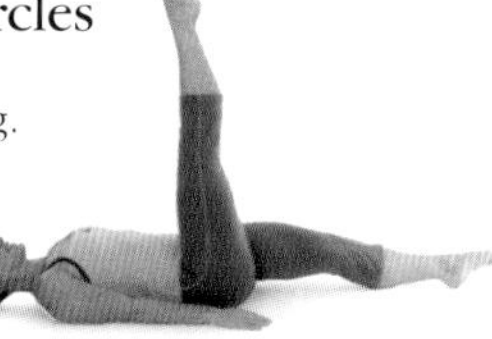

4

Rolling Like a Ball
x 5

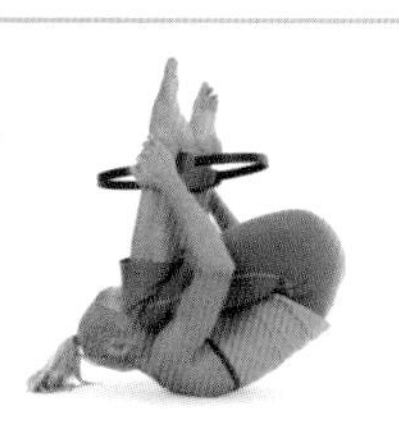

5

Stomach Series
Single-Leg Stretch x 8
Double-Leg Stretch x 8
Single-Leg Straight x 10
Double-Leg Straight x 6
Criss-Cross x 2

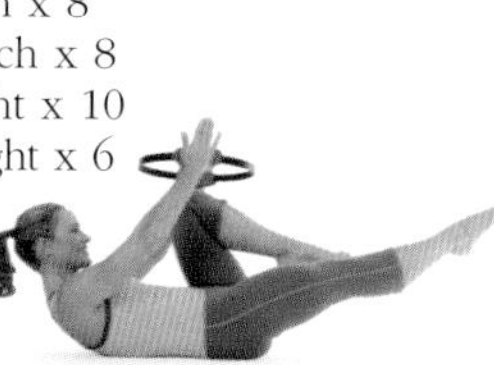

6

Spine Stretch Forward
x 3

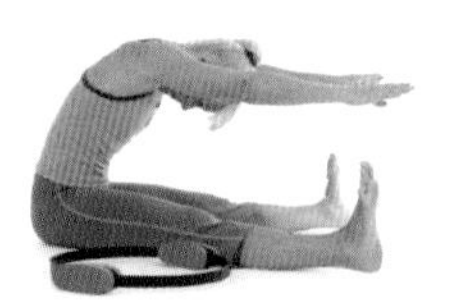

7

Open-Leg Rocker
x 5

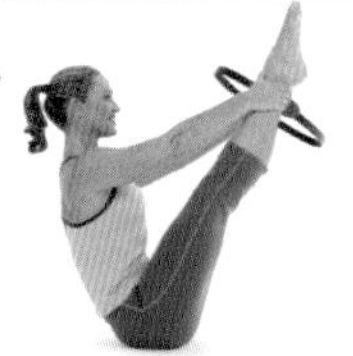

8

Corkscrew
3 sets

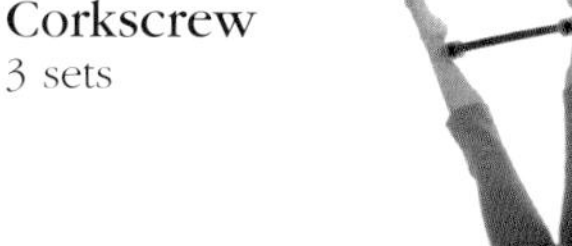

9

The Saw
3 sets

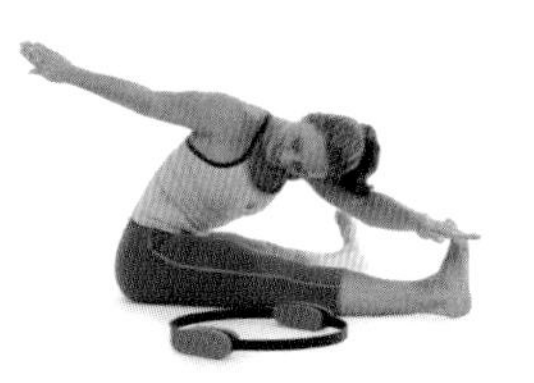

10

Prone Stomach Series
Neck Roll x 2
Single-Leg Kicks 5 sets
Double-Leg Kicks x 4

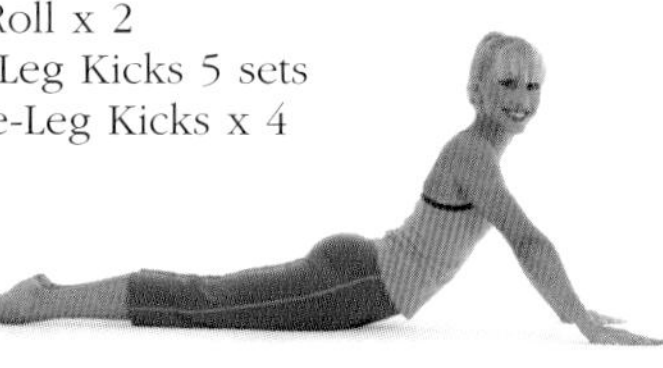

11

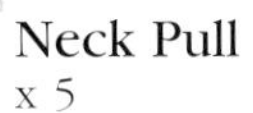

Neck Pull
x 5

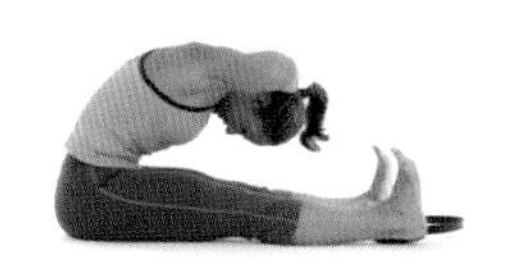

12

Side-Kick Series
Forward/Back x 8
Up/Down x 5
Small Circles
x 5 each way

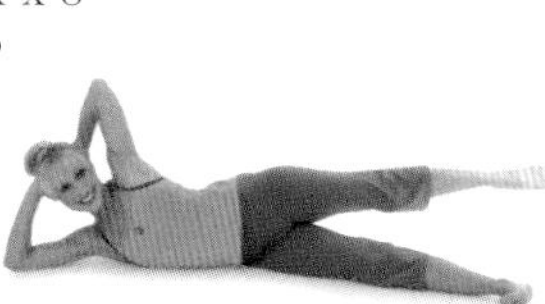

13

Lying-Leg Series
Press Down x 4
Press Up x 4
Leg Lifts
x 10 pulses

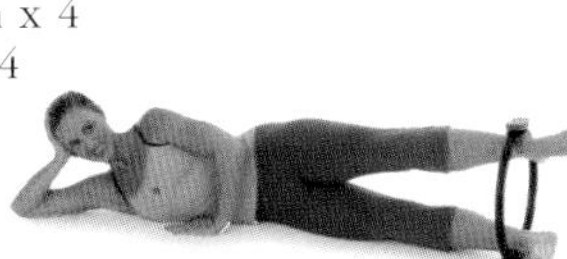

14

Transition
20 pulses

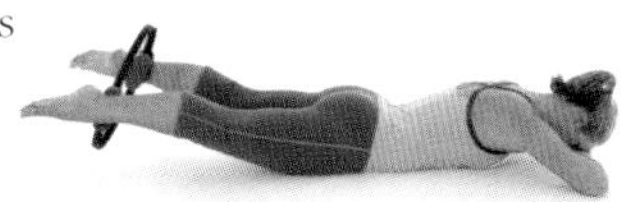

15

Teaser
Teaser Preparation 1 x 3
Teaser Preparation 2 x 2
Teaser x 3

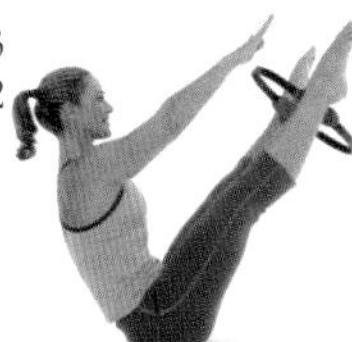

16

The Seal
x 5

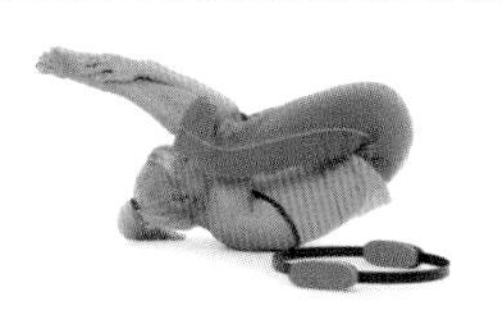

17

Push-Ups
x 3

18

Standing Arm Series
Chest x 3
Hip x 4
Head x 4
Up/Down x 2
Back hold 6 counts
Side-Arm x 3

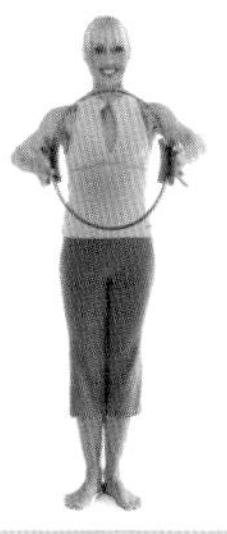

19

Standing Leg Sequence
Front x 10
Side x 10

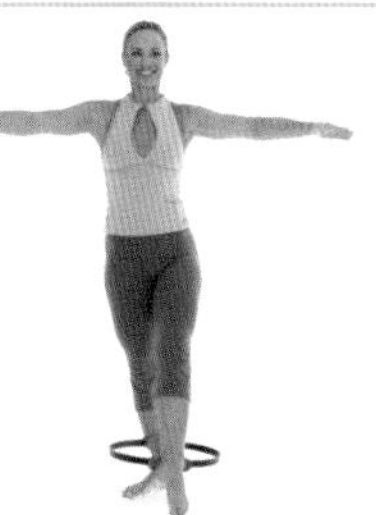

20

Seated Leg Sequence
x 6

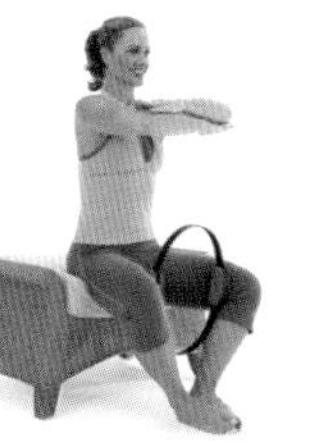

Conclusion

The more often you work through this program, the more your flexibility will increase, and your postural alignment and general body conditioning will improve.

You might discover that your arms become leaner, and stronger overall. Your legs and bottom will become firmer and more toned.

The workout circle is an extended challenge and can be integrated slowly into your workout at your own pace. Try not to add too many new exercises at once, and remember to work the mat without the workout circle for the first few times to help condition the body to an intermediate level.

To obtain the maximum benefit, remember to enforce the principles of stretch, strength and control.

If you require additional information contact Dina Matty at Pulse Health Studio, Queensland, Australia.

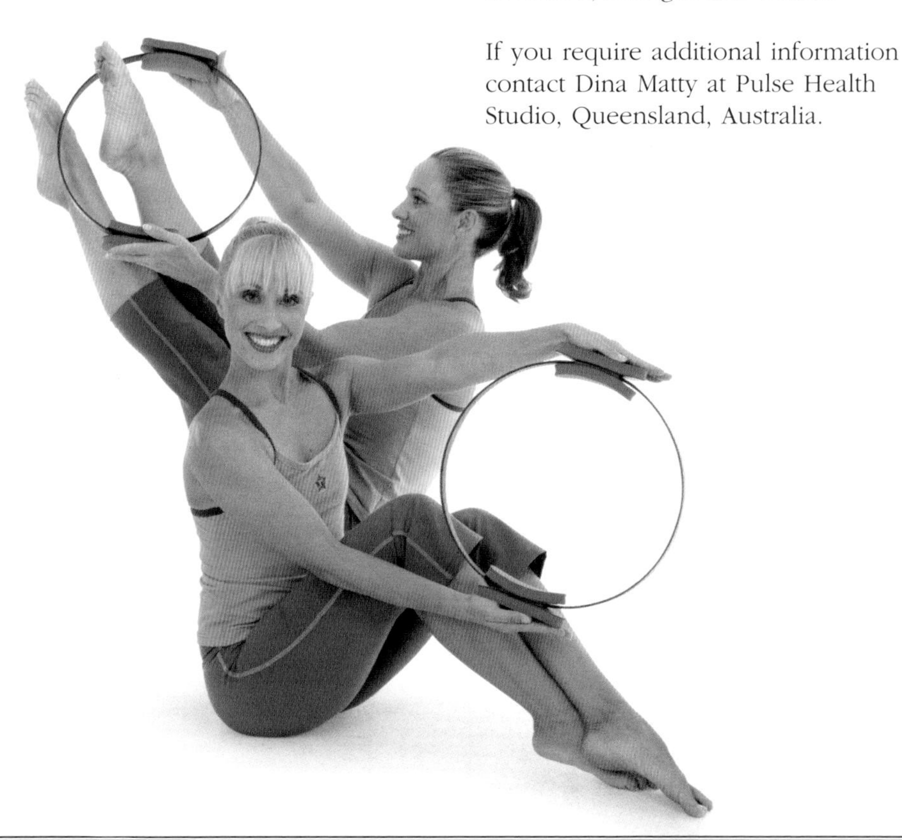

GLOSSARY

ARTICULATION
Peeling the spine segmentally down to the mat, as in the Roll-Up.

C-CURVE
The oppositional pull when you reach forward – for example in the Roll-Up, but the navel is pulled back to the spine and the torso remains curved rather than flat.

GLUTES (GLUTEUS MAXIMUS)
The largest muscle of the body; provides the bulk of the buttocks.

HAMSTRINGS
The muscle group that runs down the back of the thigh; a group of three posterior muscles working together to flex the knee and extend the thigh.

LENGTHENING
The feeling of 'growing tall', as if being pulled through the crown of the head, and extending the body through the spine.

NAVEL TO SPINE
The feeling of pulling the navel deep down internally and anchoring the back down to the mat, as if a great weight is pressing down.

PILATES STANCE
Heels together, toes splayed open to create a small 'v', wrapping the thighs around the legs and squeezing the back of the inner thighs together.

POWERHOUSE
The band of muscle about 4 cm below the navel that wraps around the torso. The powerhouse region includes the inner and outer thighs, bottom and hips.

PRONE
Lying forward, face down, on your stomach.

QUADRICEPS
The muscle group that runs down the front of the thigh. With its four parts working together, the quadriceps extends the knee and is the strongest muscle in the body.

SCOOP
The feeling of 'scooping' – internally drawing the navel in and up.

THE BOX
Two imaginary lines, one from shoulder to shoulder and the other from hip to hip.

TRICEPS
The extensor muscle at the back of the arm.

ABOUT THE AUTHORS

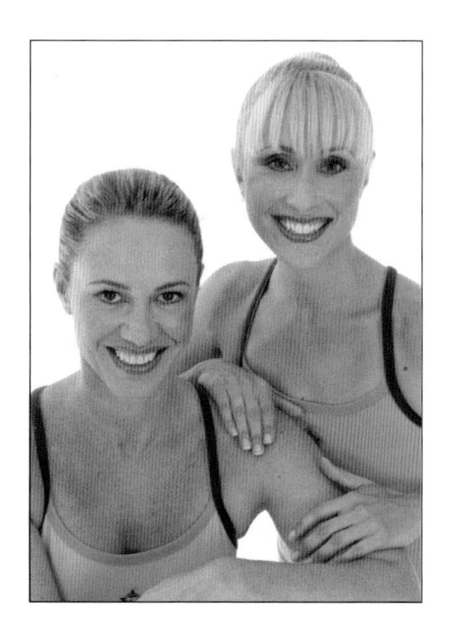

DINA MATTY *(pictured left)*
Dina is a trained dancer, aerobics champion and expert fitness teacher who studied dance in England. An exciting career in professional dancing saw Dina on television and in videos and DVDs worldwide. Taking up aerobics, Dina become the UK and European champion two years in a row. Passionate about the benefits of Pilates, Dina trained at the New York Pilates Studio in Sydney under master teachers Romana Kryzanowska and Cynthia Lochard. She is dedicated to teaching Pilates in its original format. Now in Australia, she has settled in the Gold Coast in Queensland, where she has set up Pulse Health Studio in Broadbeach.

KEFT BURDELL *(pictured right)*
Keft studied drama, movement and film at Melbourne University with a Bachelor of Education Arts. She also studied dance in the forms of classical, modern and tap. Keft combined her professional experience to become a successful personal trainer. To expand her knowledge in the fitness industry, she specialised in the field of Pilates, training at the New York Pilates Studio in Sydney, also under master trainers Romana Kryzanowska and Cynthia Lochard. Keft lives on the Gold Coast and works with Dina at Pulse Health Studio.